KU-608-922

MICHAEL McINTYRE

HERBAL MEDICINE
FOR EVERYONE

LIBRARY
WEST SUSSEX COLLEGE
OF NURSING AND MIDWIFERY
BISHOP OTTER COLLEGE
COLLEGE LANE
CHICHESTER
WEST SUSSEX PO19 4PF

ARKANA

W. SUSSEX INSTITUTE
OF
HIGHER EDUCATION
LIBRARY

ARKANA

Published by the Penguin Group
27 Wrights Lane, London W8 5TZ, England
Viking Penguin Inc., 375 Hudson Street, New York, New York 10014, USA
Penguin Books Australia Ltd, Ringwood, Victoria, Australia
Penguin Books Canada Ltd, 2801 John Street, Markham, Ontario, Canada L3R 1B4
Penguin Books (NZ) Ltd, 182–190 Wairau Road, Auckland 10, New Zealand

Penguin Books Ltd, Registered Offices: Harmondsworth, Middlesex, England

First published by Penguin Books 1988

Published by Arkana 1990
10 9 8 7 6 5 4 3 2 1

Copyright © Michael McIntyre 1988
All rights reserved

Illustrations by Sophie Allington

Printed in England by Clays Ltd, St Ives plc
Filmset in 11 on 13 pt Plantin

Except in the United States of America, this book is sold subject to
the condition that it shall not, by way of trade or otherwise, be lent,
re-sold, hired out, or otherwise circulated without the publisher's
prior consent in any form of binding or cover other than that in
which it is published and without a similar condition including this
condition being imposed on the subsequent purchaser

CONTENTS

To Annie, Zaïra and Zoë

INTRODUCTION

These are exciting times for herbalists. During the last two decades, herbal medicine, so long under the shadow of its orthodox counterpart, has begun to emerge to take its place in the sun.

The signs of this are everywhere to be seen. Seemingly overnight, whole ranges of over-the-counter herbal products have appeared on chemists' shelves. Shampoos, bath oils, soaps, cosmetics and teas trumpet their herbal origin, while supermarkets and greengrocers regularly stock a range of fresh culinary herbs to spice up their customers' diets. The back-to-nature movement is also quite apparent in a wider context. In 1974, the World Health Organization made a famous pronouncement that if the world were to achieve an adequate standard of health care by the year 2000, then Third World countries would have to nurture and develop their traditional systems of medicine rather than allow them to be supplanted by expensive modern western drugs. But developed countries which have the benefit of modern medicine have also begun to retrieve their herbal traditions. In France the first chair of herbal medicine was recently inaugurated at the University of Paris North, and French doctors queue to gain admittance to training courses in herbal medicine. In Germany a huge number of plant drug preparations (so-called phyto-pharmaceuticals) have been marketed by a large number of drug companies, and in Britain and the USA the once staunchly sceptical medical establishment has begun to take a fresh look at the herbal roots of modern medicine. Papers appear in learned medical journals on the therapeutic effects of ginseng,[1] garlic,[2] feverfew, oil of evening primrose and devil's claw,[3] to name just a few, and currently there is great interest in plants which appear to have the ability to strengthen the immune system such as echinacea and wild indigo.[4]

This unmistakable shift away from synthetic chemical medicines, cosmetics and foods in favour of those produced by nature is no doubt part of a wider 'green' revolution which increasingly demands conservation and care of our planet in place of exploitation and greed. This new planet-consciousness must, it seems, succeed, if we are to survive into the twenty-first century and beyond. Already this future is looking pretty bleak. Tropical forests, which cover around seven per cent of the earth and contain around half the planet's plant and animal species, are being decimated at a truly horrifying rate. One estimate puts the area of rain-forest being destroyed at about thirty-six thousand square miles a year (roughly the area of Holland and Switzerland combined).[5] Of the quarter of a million species of higher plants on earth only about ten per cent have been scientifically examined, usually in the most rudimentary way. What a tragedy, should this irreplaceable resource be squandered by our blind profligacy. If we change our ways, how many life-saving medicines may yet be discovered in the trees and plants of these forests?

On the positive side, the steady erosion of herbal knowledge and skills in the West due to years of neglect and derision (the reasons for which we discuss in Chapter 1) is now rapidly being reversed.

In this century, European herbal traditions survived the impact of modern western medicine and its 'magic bullets', largely due to the tenaciousness of just a few individuals, who gained their herbal training from their parents, who were herbalists before them. The famous French herbalist Maurice Mességué learnt his art from his father. In Britain, a leading figure in the world of herbal medicine, F. Fletcher

Hyde, President Emeritus of the National Institute of Medical Herbalists, whose father was also a well-known herbal practitioner, has been succeeded in practice by his two sons. In America, botanic medicine barely survived the savage onslaught of the American Medical Association. That it has done so is mainly due to the fact that it remained important to various American religious groups like the Seventh-Day Adventists and Mormons, whose doctors, like the Mormon Dr J. R. Christopher, have had considerable influence.

But in just two decades all this has changed. The growth of green-consciousness has brought forward a new breed of herbal practitioner, for the most part young men and women having no family connection with herbal medicine, but a strong and certain vocation. In the UK, this influx of highly motivated, professional herbalists made possible the resurrection of a full-time school of herbal medicine, and herbal clinics have sprung up throughout the land in most large towns and cities.

Today's herbalist, moreover, has a range of choice undreamt of by those of previous generations. In both the UK and USA alongside western-style herbalists there now work those trained in the Chinese, Ayurvedic and even Tibetan herbal traditions. In China, several of the most important traditional medical teaching hospitals now run courses (in English) to initiate practitioners into the ways of the Chinese herbalist.

Old arguments, which date back at least as far as Nicholas Culpeper, favouring indigenous herbs over imports because of their freshness and supposed relevance to local conditions, seem out of place these days when we live on imported fruit, vegetables and meat, and can travel to the other side of the earth in just a few hours. In the past, even the most traditional and conservative practitioners of herbal medicine were quick to recognize a good thing when they saw it. When, in the second half of the eighteenth century, America was being opened up by Europeans, a small supply of American ginseng (*Panax quinquelfolium*), which was well-known as a medicine to the North American Indians, found its way to China, where it was quickly recognized as an important addition to the Chinese herbal repertory. American ginseng was called *Xi yang shen* by the Chinese, literally 'western seas root'. It is interesting, however, that it was seen to be subtly different from its Chinese cousin (*Panax ginseng*). The Chinese realized that although it was not as strong (yang) as Chinese ginseng, it was a superior yin tonic. As such it had a particular application for treating tuberculosis, classic yin-deficient disease, but more generally could be used to strengthen someone in the aftermath of a high fever who showed signs of having been dried out by the fever, being weak, irritable and constantly thirsty. Chinese herb doctors could not get enough of it, and in America the 'ginseng rush' was on. American fur trappers became ginseng hunters too. One of the most famous of these trappers, Daniel Boone, actually made more money from ginseng than from all his animal pelts.[6]

Such herbal exchanges between different countries or continents were commonplace from early times. The recently republished early fifteenth-century *Mediaeval Women's Guide to Health*[7] shows that English women made use of grains of paradise, a type of cardamon and galangal (a corruption of the Chinese name, *Gao liang jiang*), both well-known in China as excellent remedies for morning sickness. Today, British herbalists would be much the poorer for the loss of a great many herbs like ginseng, ephedra, ginger, golden seal, sarsaparilla, false unicorn root and devil's claw, all imported from abroad. Moreover, there is much to be gained from comparing the way the same herbal remedies are used in different places. Sometimes there are differences. For example, while Chinese herbalists

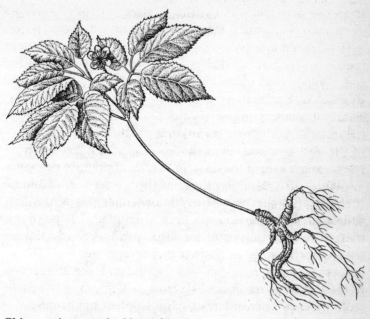

Chinese ginseng: the king of herbs

use hawthorn berries primarily as an aid to the digestion, in the West these berries are chiefly used as a heart tonic, also being good for helping to regulate blood pressure. Mugwort in the western tradition has emmenagogic properties (i.e. the ability to bring on a delayed period), but in the Chinese tradition, where a woman is deficient and cold (see Appendix B), it is actually used to stop menstrual bleeding and can be used to treat some cases of threatened miscarriage. For the most part, however, a comparison of the same herbs used by different traditions shows remarkable unanimity, which must strengthen the case for the efficacy of herbal medicine in the absence of modern scientific investigation.

Such comparisons are a feature of this book, which sets out to give a picture of the modern herbalist at work, both from the herbalist's and patient's perspective. Although a great many allopathic drugs derive from plant medicines, herbal medicine is essentially different from modern medicine. Its plant remedies and style are holistic, treating the whole person rather than concentrating on any specific disease. Its methods have been tried and tested over thousands of years, without recourse to cruel animal experimentation. Aside from comparing the different approaches of the herbalist and the orthodox doctor, I have also tried to give some idea of the different styles of practice currently available – for example, those of the western and Chinese herbalist. To the best of my knowledge, this is the first time such a comparison has been attempted. I hope that it will prove a starting point for subsequent work of a similar nature, for it is my belief that the development and future success of herbal medicine will depend on some integration of these various traditional systems, which can only benefit from modern scientific research into plant medicines.

We herbalists have much to learn from each other and much to offer the community. Some years ago, I had the opportunity to work for a few months in a Chinese hospital of traditional medicine, which was staffed entirely by herbal and acupuncture doctors. It was a fascinating experience, for these traditional doctors showed themselves highly competent to treat a wide range of diseases, some of which, like appendicitis, would only be treated by surgery in the West. The 'drug trolley' bearing medications around the hospital wards I worked in was a sight to behold, for it was packed with thermos flasks filled with individual prescribed herbal decoctions, each one destined for patients who would drink it throughout the day. The hospital pharmacy was a large room, the walls of which were lined floor to ceiling with wooden drawers containing a great assortment of dried roots and herbs, from which the pharmacists would make a selection according to a prescription, which would then be deftly folded into a paper packet to be given to the patient to take home and drink as a decoction.

Could such sights be seen in our modern, high-tech hospitals? The idea might seem ludicrous, but I believe that herbal and modern medicine can work well alongside one another. Such a blend of old and new can be seen in China and India, where western-medicine hospitals commonly trade patients with the traditional-medicine hospitals. If herbal medicine were to be more widely available here, it would contribute enormously to health-care and disease prevention in this country, and wipe millions off the NHS drug bill. In espousing modern medicine to the exclusion of alternative systems of medicine, we have, I think, thrown the baby out with the bath water. But the situation is one of flux and change, and I predict that it will not be long before herbal treatment will once again be as acceptable and commonplace as it once was, albeit in a form more suited to twentieth-century needs.

> And the end of all our exploring
> Will be to arrive where we started
> And know the place for the first time.

> T. S. Eliot *Little Gidding*

CHAPTER ONE

HISTORY

Plants have been synonymous with medicine since the beginning of time. Moreover, their medicinal use is common to all cultures and peoples of the world. Just how revered and ancient herbal medicine is, is implied by several biblical references like that of Ecclesiasticus 38:4, 'The Lord hath created medicines out of the earth', and Psalm 104:14, 'He [God] causeth herbs to grow for the service of man.'

The Book of Enoch, an ancient Ethiopian text written some time between the second and first centuries B C, in a remarkable development of the mysterious passage in the sixth chapter of Genesis, likewise specifically credits human discovery of herbal medicine to the gods themselves: 'Sons of God' took to themselves 'wives of the daughters of men' and these 'angels, sons of heaven' taught their wives 'medicines and incantations, and the cuttings of roots and plants they made known unto them'.[1]

This fascinating ancient story, which would make women the first human herbalists, is in keeping with the facts of later history, for some of the greatest herbalists have been women. Modern medicine can be thankful for many so-called old wives' secrets handed down through the generations.*

---

* It was just such a grandmother's secret that led to the discovery of the drug digitalis, now usually used as digoxin or lanoxin in the treatment of heart disease all over the world. In 1775 a young doctor, William Withering, was asked to cure a case of dropsy (an accumulation of fluid in the tissues). He described what followed. 'I was told that it [the cure] had long been kept a secret by an old woman in Shropshire, who had made cures after the more regular practitioners had failed ... It was not difficult ... to perceive that the active herb could be none other than Foxglove [*Digitalis purpurea*].'[2]

No matter which culture one explores, the theme that the first herbalists were part human, part gods, is evident. In China, Huang Di, the legendary and god-like Yellow Emperor, is credited with the authorship of *The Yellow Emperor's Classic of Internal Medicine* (*Huang-di Nei-Jing*). He is also said to have invented the chariot, coinage, musical notation and woven the first clothing. His reign began around 2697 BC, but the *Classic of Internal Medicine* was in fact almost certainly compiled much later, between 200 and 100 BC by several authors. Even so, it is still the oldest extant major Chinese medical text, in which are listed thirteen herbal prescriptions.

The Yellow Emperor's predecessor, a similarly mythical figure, called Shen Nong, whose reign ended as that of the Yellow Emperor began, is said to have compiled the *Shen Nong Ben Cao* (*Shen Nong's Materia Medica*). According to legend, this Emperor must have been just as busy as the Yellow Emperor, for, in addition to inventing the plough and animal husbandry, he found time to explore the marshes, forests and fields, tasting for himself 'the hundred herbs'. Chinese herbalists still tell the story how, in pursuit of his herbal art, the Emperor Shen Nong poisoned himself eighty times a day, but such was his skill with plant medicines that he always found an antidote. Small wonder, in view of his dedication, that in China he is revered as the patron of herbal medicine. The truth, however, is again somewhat more prosaic, for the *Shen Nong*, which means literally 'divine farmer', was put together no earlier than the first century BC, again in all probability by several authors. Even in these early times people evidently felt the need to invoke the distant past to lend authority to their works. This too is a recurring theme in the development of herbal medicine, giving it a markedly different viewpoint from that of modern medicine, where a textbook is generally out-of-date a year or two after its publication.

Similar mythology shrouds the origins of herbal medicine in the West, which looks back to ancient Egypt for its roots. The Egyptians were the most renowned of all ancient peoples for their skill with herbs. The Greek historian Herodotus writes of an inscription inside the Great Pyramid at Gisa, which tells that quantities of garlic, onions and radishes were consumed by the workers building the pyramids, presumably to strengthen their resolve and up their productivity.

Imhotep, chief architect to King Zozer, was to the ancient Egyptians the counterpart of Emperor Shen Nong in China, for he is reputed to have set down on paper (actually papyrus, of course) an authoritative 'book' of herbal medicine. Sadly, if this treatise did exist, it has long since been destroyed. However, the Egyptians were well-acquainted with most of the herbs we find mentioned in the *Ebers Papyrus*,[3] written many centuries earlier in 1500 BC, for official schools of herbalists existed in Egypt as early as 3000 BC.

The *Ebers Papyrus*, discovered in an ancient tomb in 1862, contains references to more than 700 herbal remedies, including aloes, caraway seeds, castor oil and squill, while some of its recipes, like this hairwash for Queen Shesh of Egypt, would hardly be likely to make the beauty pages of today's fashion magazines:

> The claw of a dog
> Decayed palm leaves ⎬ in equal parts
> The hoof of an ass

Boil thoroughly in oil and rub on to the head.

Others are more familiar:

> To stop diarrhoea
> Spring onions
> Groats recently boiled

Oil and honey
Wax and water
Boil together and drink for four days.

When we read these ancient prescriptions we should do so with an open mind. Toothache was believed to be caused by a worm attacking the tooth, and the following incantation from an ancient Assyrian herbal was used to drive it out.

After Anu made the heavens, the heavens made the earth.
The earth made the rivers, the rivers the canals,
The canals the marsh, the marsh made the worm,
The worm came weeping to Shamash,
Came to Ea, her tears flowing.
'What wilt thou give me for my food,
What wilt thou give me to destroy?'
'I will give thee dried figs and apricots.'
'Forsooth, what are these dried figs to me or apricots?
Set me amid the teeth and let me dwell in the gums,
That I may destroy the blood of the teeth and of the gums chew their marrow.'
'Since thou has said this, oh worm,
May Ea smite thee with his mighty fist.'[4]

The idea that disease, particularly toothache, could be caused by a worm was prevalent throughout early and mediaeval Europe. We find it mentioned, for example, in the Anglo-Saxon herbal *The Leech Book of Bald*. But is this apparently naïve idea so far removed from modern knowledge that microscopic bacteria can cause infection and tooth decay?

The great Assyrian herbal, from which this incantation comes, has come down to us in some 40,000 fragments of stone tablets, found among the ruins of the Great Library of the Temples at Nineveh. Painstaking scholarship has demonstrated that when complete it contains the Assyrian and Sumerian names of around a thousand plants, showing that the names by which we know many plants today are derived from the ancient Sumerian language through Greek and Arabic. When we use words like saffron, carob, cardamom, cumin, turmeric, cherry, flax, myrrh, mulberry, mandrake, almond, poppy, sesame, cypress and lupin, it turns out that we are actually speaking a distant dialect of ancient Sumerian.

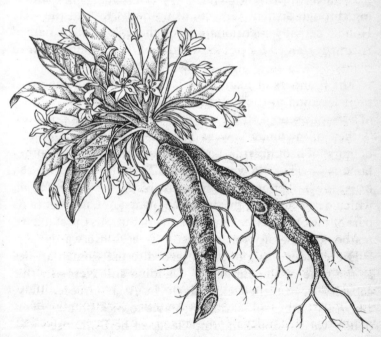

Mandrake was used in Roman times as an anaesthetic.

The medical inheritance of ancient Egypt passed to Greece, to Rome, and thence to the Arabs. The Greeks, like the Egyptians, also believed that the gods were the first herbalists and physicians. Perhaps because they recognized their debt to the ancient Egyptian medical schools, the Greeks identified their god of medicine, Asclepius, with the Egyptian god-healer Imhotep, whom the Greeks said emigrated to Greece from Memphis in Egypt to reside at Epidaurus. According to the Greeks, Asclepius was none other than the son of Apollo, the sun god, who was taught his art by Cheiron, and whose daughter was Hygeia (from whom we inherit our word hygiene), the goddess of health.

As well as priests at the temple of Asclepius, many lay herb-doctors called Asclepiadae earned their living wandering through ancient Greece, using herbs to heal the sick. Homer actually mentions one of these, a woman named Agamede, famed for her knowledge of the healing power of plants.

The founders of many Greek schools of medicine owed their learning to the Egyptians. Both Pythagoras, founder of a famous school on the island of Samos, and Hippocrates, 'father of medicine', were tutored by Egyptian priest-doctors. Theophrastus and Dioscorides were two other famous Greeks who wrote herbals. Theophrastus (372–285 BC) is the 'father of botany' because his *Historia Plantarum*, which describes over five hundred plants, not only contains part of the oldest Greek herbal known, but was the standard textbook on botany for hundreds of years afterwards.

Dioscorides was a doctor attached to the Roman armies at the time of the Emperors Claudius and Nero. In this capacity he travelled extensively in Asia, Greece, Italy, Germany and Gaul, and so was able to pick up a tremendously varied, first-hand knowledge of herbs. Dioscorides compiled all the contemporary herbal knowledge in his book *De Materia Medica*, which set a pattern for professional herbals thereafter. For more than thirteen centuries it was one of the principal medical textbooks throughout the civilized world. Even in the nineteenth century it was still in use in the Turkish empire.

The Greek herbal achieved its final form in the work of Claudius Galen, who was born around AD 130. He was physician to the Roman Emperor and philosopher Marcus Aurelius and was himself famous as a healer, teacher and philosopher. His herbal, *De Simplicibus*, was used by the Arabs along with other Greek herbals and formed the basis of the medical school at Cairo, directed by the famous Arab botanist Abdullah Ibn Al-Baitar in 1248. The Arabs were able to draw not only on Greek and Egyptian teaching, but also on the ancient Ayurvedic (Indian) and Persian traditions.

We know little about the herbal medicine of pre-Roman Britain. The esteem in which the Celtic people held plants may be gathered from the famous story of the mistletoe under which we still kiss, pagan fashion, at Christmas time. Mistletoe was greatly revered by the Druids. It had to be culled from an oak tree (where it grows only rarely) and could only be cut down with a golden sickle. Mistletoe is propagated by fruit-eating birds like thrushes and wax-wings, which wipe their beaks free of the sticky pulp in which the seeds lie, against a branch of a tree or spread the seed to other trees through their droppings. The plant never touches the ground, since it roots in the parent tree as it grows. For this reason it was seen as a celestial plant; being rooted in an earthly tree it was thought to have the power to intercede on behalf of heaven, unifying the energy of heaven and earth. If the mistletoe touched the ground, it was thought by the Druids that misfortune would befall the nation.

It is fascinating to think that so many centuries later, a modern Swiss anti-cancer pharmaceutical preparation called Ischador formulated by Rudolf Steiner, which contains mistletoe, is made by observing similar con-

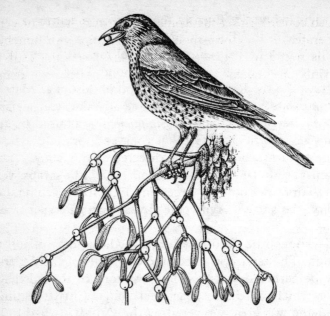

Mistlethrush on mistletoe

straints. The mistletoe used in this herbal drug is never allowed to touch anything inorganic during the manufacturing process. Steiner and his anthroposophical medical school consider this necessary to preserve the full healing power of the herb.*

The Romans who colonized Britain in the first century AD found the country unbearably cold and damp after sunny Italy. We know this because the legionaries brought with them many Mediterranean herbs like rosemary, oregano and the seeds of an Italian variety of the common nettle (*Urtica pilulifera*), whose sting is far stronger than its

---

* A recent study in *Oncology*[5] reported research concerning twenty patients with breast cancer who received a single intravenous dose of Ischador. The patients showed a favourable reaction following a pattern 'similar to that which has been described after treatment with Interferon'. (Interferon is an anti-viral substance, naturally produced in response to infection with a virus.)

British cousin. Either the Romans were very hardy or very desperate, for they beat their arthritic limbs with bunches of this nettle to alleviate the pain and swelling. This is certainly one ancient treatment you will not receive at the hands of a modern herbalist!

The oldest Saxon herbal we still have is *The Leech Book of Bald*. Leech is an old name for doctor. Despite being over 1,000 years old, it is still in good condition. It was much valued by generations of monks, like those at Glastonbury where it was kept, who tended their gardens and the sick with its help.

The *Leech Book* shows that Anglo-Saxons used a far larger number of herbs than their contemporaries in Europe. Their herbal remedies were mixed with honey, ale and vinegar. Ointments were made with honey. Their favourite herbs were betony, vervain and plantain, which they called waybroad. When you think about Anglo-Saxon history, it is not surprising that many of the remedies are for broken heads and bleeding noses.

The vast repository of herbal know-how of the ancient world which had been lost to Europe in the 'dark ages' filtered back (as did much other vital knowledge) through the Crusaders returning from the Middle East, and was safely 'housed' in the walled gardens of monasteries throughout Europe. The monks, a major part of whose work was the care of the sick, were skilled copyists, and until the invention of printing were probably the most important source of herbal books. It is from this period that many of the great monastic tonic remedies which we now drink as liqueurs were invented. The original medicinal properties of such tipples as benedictine or chartreuse are, alas, long since lost, but even now their formulae are closely guarded and treasured secrets. Today, only two monks at any one time from La Grande Chartreuse, near Grenoble, are permitted to know the secret herbal ingredients of the liqueur that has made their monastery a household name throughout the world.

With the advent of printing came widespread dissemination of herbal knowledge. No doubt thoroughly alarmed by this boom in herbal medicine, rich and influential doctors at the Court of Henry VIII put pressure on the King to protect their privileged position; in 1511 the King sought to prevent any physician practising 'except he first be examined by the Bishop of London or Dean of St Paul's calling to him four doctors physic'.

But the new law brought about an intolerable situation, for there were not enough doctors to go round, even if the common people could have afforded their treatment, which they certainly could not. As a result in 1543, in a famous law now known as the Herbalist's Charter, Henry VIII reversed his decision and gave rights to all his subjects to practise herbal medicine.

Be it ordained, established and enacted by authority of this present Parliament, that at all time from henceforth, it shall be lawful to every person, being the King's subject, having knowledge and experience of the nature of Herbs, Roots and Waters . . . within any part of the realm of England, or within any other of the King's dominions, to practise, use and minister in and to any Outward Sore, Uncome Wound, Apostemations, Outward Swelling or Disease any Herb or Herbs, Ointments, Baths, Pulters and Emplaisters, according to their Cunning, Experience and Knowledge in any of the Diseases, Sores or Maladies aforesaid, and all other like to the same, or Drinks for the Stone, Stranguary, or Agues, without Suit, Vexation, Trouble, Penalty or Loss of their Goods.

If Henry VIII said it was all right, no one was going to argue! Now herbal medicine was free to flourish and the Elizabethan era saw the publication of many famous herbals. William Turner's *New Herball*, published in 1551, was dedicated to Elizabeth I. Turner was the first

Englishman to study plants scientifically, and like Theophrastus before him, is called the 'father of botany'. The herbals of this time are worth reading as much for their social commentary as for their medicine. The streets of Elizabethan London must have been hazardous to health. Turner prescribes walnuts 'for the bytings of both men and doggs'.

Perhaps the most famous English herbal of all was that of John Gerard, herbalist to James I. Gerard had a garden in Fetter Lane, London, where he grew more than a thousand varieties of herbs, including the first potatoes brought back from the New World by Sir Walter Raleigh. His herbal, published in 1597, was largely drawn from a herbal by the Dutchman Dodoens and describes around two thousand plants.

But despite the printing of many other popular herbals, like John Parkinson's *Paradisi in Sole* (*Park in the Sun*) – a pun on the author's name – published in 1629, by the beginning of the eighteenth century herbal medicine had begun to fall out of favour with the medical profession.

The reasons for this are complex but traceable. Today this break with the past is often said to be due to the unscientific beliefs which herbalists held – in particular the 'doctrine of signatures' and the mixing of astrology with herbal medicine.

The doctrine of signatures was the belief that plants carried a sign or signature denoting their medicinal properties. Adherents of the doctrine pointed to such examples as the root tubers of pilewort, which they said resembled haemorrhoids, and so used the plant for this complaint (it is still a useful remedy for piles), or to the flowers of skullcap, in which they discerned the shape of the human skull and hence used this plant to treat headaches. Crudely applied in this way, the idea seems nothing short of banal and certainly it was taken to ludicrous lengths, but the essential idea that the healing nature of a plant might be discerned by its taste (see Chapter 2) or pattern of growth may not be so far-fetched. Indeed it is to the doctrine of signatures that modern medicine owes one of its most famous drugs, for in 1763 it led the Reverend Edward Stone to investigate the medicinal property of willow bark. Stone noticed that willows grew in marshy regions where rheumatism was common, and decided to try out a decoction of the bark on sufferers of the disease. To his delight, this old folk remedy proved itself reliable, a fact which science subsequently confirmed when, three-quarters of a century later, salicylic acid – or in other words, aspirin – was extracted from willow bark.

As for astrology, its main proponent, Nicholas Culpeper, is now often blamed for bringing herbal medicine into disrepute by prescribing plants according to the astrological signs to which they were attributed. Culpeper was a flamboyant, revolutionary figure, whose studies at Cambridge were abruptly curtailed after a disastrous and abortive attempt at elopement with a young heiress (on the way to join her lover she was killed when lightning struck her coach). Abandoning his former way of life, Culpeper was apprenticed to an apothecary in London and was soon practising medicine himself. Full of scorn for the supercilious and money-grabbing behaviour of many of the doctors of his time, he soon incurred the wrath of the medical establishment by daring to translate the Latin pharmacopoeia into English for all to read. He also went out on a limb by treating the poor free of charge. But in his interest in astrology Culpeper was anything but revolutionary, since it was considered a perfectly respectable study by his contemporaries. Sir Isaac Newton, for instance, writing a few years after Culpeper's death, devoted a large number of his later works to the 'science' of astrology.

Other factors, then, were responsible for undermining the practice of herbal medicine as it had been known since the time of Hippocrates and Galen. The time was ripe for change because of the ultra-conservatism of the European schools, which insisted that their students should regurgitate line for line in Greek and Latin the works of these ancient Greek doctors. The Paris medical school in the seventeenth century was typical: the head professor admonished his students, 'Read only Hippocrates, Galen and Aristotle ... learn by heart the aphorisms of Hippocrates.'[6]

Such a stick-in-the-mud attitude invited revolt, and it came in the form of a larger-than-life character, Philippus Theophrastus Bombastus von Hohenheim, who, claiming to be an alchemist, called himself Paracelsus. Paracelsus displayed total scorn for the old ways. He publicly burnt the books of Hippocrates and Galen, threw aside their ideas and introduced to internal medicine chemical preparations of such minerals as arsenic, sulphur, lead, copper, iron, silver, gold, mercury and antimony.

Paracelsus' revolution went beyond his new *Materia Medica*, for he argued that individual preparations could be used to treat specific diseases. Because of this he has been unfairly blamed for abandoning holistic medicine. But in many ways he was a traditional herbalist who insisted on throwing out the mumbo-jumbo that had accumulated through the years, substituting instead his own hard-won clinical experience. Moreover, he probably only used metals in tiny amounts, more akin to the practices of homeopathy than allopathy, for, as Barbara Griggs points out in her excellent *Green Pharmacy*,

Paracelsus' advocacy of mineral poisons like mercury and antimony, which has been seen as one of the most distinctive contributions to the evolution of medicine, is, in fact, based on a belief common in Swiss-German medicine at the time – and three centuries later to become famous as homeopathy – that like is cured by like, the effects of poison remedied by doses of another poison.[7]

As Paracelsus himself wrote, 'It depends only upon the dose whether a poison is a poison or not.'[8]

If we are to blame anyone for abandoning the holistic approach, it should be those who followed Paracelsus, who paid no heed to his dictum and used poisonous metals internally in dangerous doses, concentrating on treating the disease rather than the patient – a fundamental change of outlook which was coincidentally encouraged by the discovery of herbal remedies from America which gained an extraordinary reputation for the treatment of specific diseases.

Thus Peruvian bark (*Cinchona succirubra*) was found to be a sure-fire cure for malaria, and ipecac (*Cephaelis ipecacuanha*) useful for treating dysentery, while guaiac (*Guaiacum officinale*) and sarsaparilla (*Smilax ornata*) were held to be specific for syphilis, which was a terrifying scourge, just as AIDS has become today. These herbs and their metallic counterparts (mercury for syphilis, for instance) and the fact that doctors became interested in finding a cure for each disease rather than in trying to treat the whole patient, meant that the use of poisonous metals and plants swept the gentler herbal remedies from the pharmacopeias. John Waller commented on this trend in his *New British Domestic Herbal* published in 1822:

Advantages have accrued to medicine from chemical preparations; it is nevertheless a melancholy truth that the health of thousands and the lives of not a few are yearly sacrificed to the rage for preparations of mercury, arsenic and almost every deleterious mineral under heaven. So far has this rage for poisonous drugs gained ground that scarcely any article from the plant kingdom is thought worthy to enter into the prescription of a modern physician, that is not recognized for a dangerous and active poison, hence the daily use of aconite, hemlock, henbane, etc.

These radical changes in the world of medicine were, of course, part of a much greater and more profound revolution which we call the birth of the scientific age. When Copernicus discovered that the world was not, after all, at the centre of the universe, the vacuum this created in contemporary cosmology was filled not by the sun but by the human mind. The French writer, Rabelais, identified the new attitude when he cheekily re-wrote St Augustine's advice, 'Love and do as you will', merely as 'Do as you will'. Scientific discoveries of the eighteenth and nineteenth centuries seemed to confirm that there were no limits to what mankind could achieve through measurement and experiment. This science was youthful and brash and it overturned and trampled on the old order. Medical advances like William Harvey's discovery of the way the blood circulated ousted the ancient ideas of humours and herbs, which seemed far too imprecise. The new science of pharmacology reacted against the 'inexactitudes' of herbal preparations by isolating and finally synthesizing active principles from medicinal plants so that it was no longer necessary to have recourse to the vagaries of nature. Thus the famous heart drug, digitalis, was extracted from the foxglove, aspirin from the willow bark, reserpine from the Indian plant rauwolfia, steroids from the Mexican yam, and so on.

From this time onwards herbal medicine was all but obscured under the shadow of modern scientific medicine. In Britain, professional herbal medicine survived only through the birth in 1864 of the National Association of Medical Herbalists, which is flourishing today under the name of the National Institute of Medical Herbalists.

The original inspiration for this body came from America where an important school of herbal medicine called physiomedicalism had many practitioners at the end of the nineteenth century. The physiomedical herbal doctors blended both traditional British herbal lore brought to the USA by the pilgrim fathers with that of the North American Indians. The founder of this system of medicine was Samuel Thomson (1769–1843), famous for his rediscovery of an ancient North American Indian remedy, Lobelia. Thomson never went to school, but instead helped to gather plants for a local herbalist. He encountered the herb medicines and healing principles of the North American Indian natives, which essentially resembled the classical ideas of natural healing which had been practised by herbalists in Europe and Asia for thousands of years. Thomson advocated that the body should be cleansed by elimination of waste materials. His idea of steaming the body, which the American settlers saw in the North American Indian sweat lodges, had also been practised by the Russians and Turks for centuries. At a time when orthodox medicine used blood-letting to treat every disease and administered violent purgatives and poisons, Thomson revived ancient and profound concepts of healing, essentially relying on the body's own healing power, and insisting that the herbalist's job was only to help and never to interfere with this process.

Thomson met with enormous opposition from the orthodox doctors. They actually persuaded the New Hampshire legislature to pass a bill forbidding him by name to treat people for any ailment.

Today these ideas of natural healing are as controversial and important as they ever were, for although the value of modern medicine in coping with acute or life-threatening disease is plain to see, modern drugs are entirely disease-orientated. Allopathic medicine in its bid to conquer disease

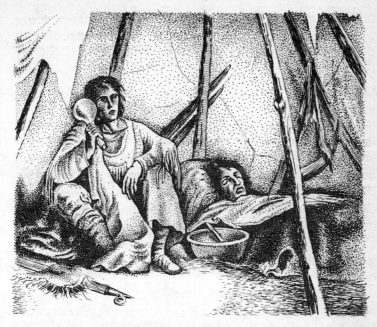

White settlers learnt North American Indian herbal medicine from the medicine men, whose mortar and pestle for mixing medicines still is, a familiar tool in pharmacies.

has in some strange way apparently lost sight of the human beings who are ill, and of the subtle emotional, mental and physical factors that can determine whether someone is healthy or ill. The powerful drugs it uses have many unwanted side-effects and are not suitable tools for redressing the imbalances that underlie chronic degenerative diseases, nor indeed for promoting the prevention of disease. In these respects herbal medicine has much to offer.

I would suggest that the whole imposing edifice of modern medicine, for all its breathtaking successes, is, like the celebrated Tower of Pisa, slightly off balance. No one could be stupid enough to deny the enormous benefits which the advances of medical science in this century have conferred upon us all ... but, nevertheless, the fact remains that contemporary medicine as a whole tends to be fascinated by the objective, statistical, computerized approach to healing the sick.

If disease is regarded as an objective problem isolated from all personal factors then surgery plus more and more powerful drugs must be the answer ... It is frightening how dependent upon drugs we are becoming and how easy it is for doctors to present them as the universal panacea for our ills. Wonderful as many of them are, it should be more widely stressed by doctors that the health of human beings is so often determined by their behaviour, their food and the nature of their environment.

Prince Charles. Extract of speech
to the BMA on the occasion of its 150th anniversary
December 1982.

CHAPTER TWO

PRINCIPLES

Herbal medicine differs from many other systems of alternative medicine because, as we have seen, it does not belong to any one culture, nor is it the inspiration of any one person. Acupuncture, on the other hand, has a unique philosophy and methodology which is unmistakably Chinese. Homeopathy, the brain-child of Samuel Hahnemann, is claimed to be a complete and quite distinct system of medicine, with an integrated philosophy based on the principle of 'like curing like'. But when one surveys the range and variety of herbal treatment throughout the ages and from culture to culture, it may seem there exists no cogent theme or philosophy, no guiding hand or spirit behind the practice of it.

Such a view may well be reinforced by the flurry of recently published books on herbal medicine which suggest that a single herb can be used to treat a huge list of diseases or symptoms. Is this really all there is to herbal medicine? Is it merely symptomatic, mimicking with plants what orthodox medicine does with drugs? Happily, a closer inspection of the many different ways herbal medicine has been practised does show that there are indeed common underlying holistic themes and methods of practice that are as relevant to the twentieth century as they always have been.

Surveying the landscape of herbal practice, one may discern at least four quite distinct forms or methods of prescribing herbs and the modern herbalist can be heir to all of them.

The first 'method' is the most difficult for us to understand because by definition it lies outside or beyond logical thought processes. We might describe this type of plant therapy as entirely instinctive or intuitive herbalism. It can be seen amongst sick animals when they display an uncanny ability to search out healing plants. Several herbs, for this reason, were named after the animals which used them as medicines. When off-colour a dog or cat will eat couch grass, also known as dog's grass, to induce vomiting and rid the system of toxins. Greater celandine (*Chelidonium majus*) derives its name from the Greek word for a swallow – χελιδών – because in ancient times it was believed that swallows would rub a sprig of this plant on the eyes of their young to open them. The French herbalist Maurice Mességué says that his father actually saw this happen. And if this seems far-fetched consider the following recent report about the behaviour of African chimpanzees:

Chimpanzees in the wild appear to practise herbal medicine. Moreover, according to scientists who have observed this behaviour, the leaves that the chimps methodically seek out and swallow, apparently when ill, contain a substance that shows promise as a drug for humans.

The leaves from a bushy plant called Aspilia contain a substance that laboratory studies show to be a potent killer of bacteria, fungi and nematodes, all of which can cause serious disease in apes and humans alike ... At Gombe (Tanzania's National Park), chimps seek out the leaves as soon as they wake up in the morning. Instead of breakfasting at the nearest source of wild fruit, which is their usual practice, some chimps will walk for twenty minutes or more to open, grassy areas where Aspilia grows.

Instead of promptly tearing off the leaves and eating them, the animal gingerly closes its lips over the unplucked leaf and holds it for a few seconds. Several leaves are tried in this way before the chimp selects one and places it in its mouth. Instead of chewing, the ape rolls the leaf around its mouth for perhaps fifteen seconds and then swallows it whole.

Chimp researchers have long speculated on the role of the leaves ... Part of the answer emerged last year. Eloy Rodriguez, a biochemist at the University of California – Irvine, began searching for unusual chemicals in Aspilia leaves and quickly isolated a previously unknown substance, a red oil later named thiarubrine-A ... a powerful antibiotic capable of killing common disease-causing bacteria in concentrations of less than one part per million.[1]

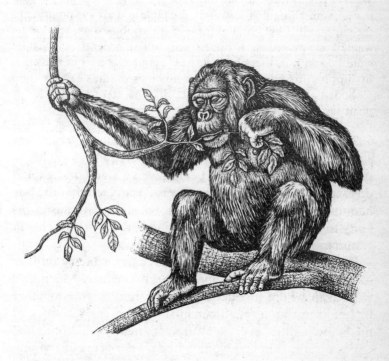

We humans also display a similar instinctive ability. Many people experience a desire for citrus fruit, such as oranges, when they have a cold (the vitamin C citrus fruit contain reinforces the immune system to combat a cold). Such an instinct is often heightened in pregnant women, who may crave strange and exotic foods, perhaps because they are depleted of some vitamin or mineral which that food will supply. This instinctual wisdom is also often alive in young children, whose natural responses have not yet been conditioned into submission. A striking and sad example of this was recorded in the city of Baltimore. A young boy had a craving for salt. His mother told the doctor what happened when the child was eighteen months old . . .

When I would feed him his dinner at noon, he would keep crying out for something that wasn't on the table and always pointing to the cupboard. I held him in front of the cupboard to see what he wanted. He picked out the salt at once and in order to see what he would do with it, I let him have it. He poured some out and ate it by dipping his finger in it. After this he wouldn't eat any food without having salt too. It seemed like he ate a terrible lot of plain salt.

The unhappy end to this story was that the child was subsequently admitted to hospital, where he was unable to satisfy his craving for salt, being given a standard hospital diet, and he died. Afterwards it was discovered that the boy had suffered an adrenal-gland imbalance that caused his body to be deficient in sodium – one of the two elements in common salt.

But these examples only hint at the extraordinary abilities of the first herbalists whom we call Shamans: men and women in whom instinct has been raised to an altogether higher intuitive level. Shamanism is the early history of medicine within every culture. In nearly all aboriginal tribes certain men and women underwent years of training to develop in themselves an inner eye, which enabled them to become seers and to communicate directly with the plant world during the practice of their healing art. As Richard Grossinger puts it in his book *Planet Medicine*: 'Early human experimenters tried to get back inside Nature so they could hear her original voice.'[2] A pueblo Indian chief explained more simply: 'Plants too were living beings; we talked to them and if the words were genuine, the plants talked back.'

To attain the necessary visionary state, Shamans would often make use of hallucinogenic plants, which have been used throughout the world for this purpose. In this we hear echoes of *The Book of Enoch* (see Chapter 1), for all aboriginal societies considered, and still do, that plants like *Soma*, the ancient God-narcotic of India, or the sacred Mexican mushrooms which the Aztecs called *teonanactl* ('divine flesh'), were gifts of the gods and were to be treated with the greatest reverence.

A modern account of Shamanism is given by Carlos Castaneda in his vivid description of his training with the Yaqui Indian Don Juan. His stories are so striking because they are an account from the inside – a glimpse of another world; a separate reality and a kind of herbalism that is altogether beyond our mundane knowledge:

Don Juan said that he had used power plants to shake my assemblage point out of its normal setting. The effect of power plants is much like that of dreams. Dreams make the assemblance point move, but power plants manage the shift on a greater and more engulfing scale. A teacher then uses the disorientating effects of such a shift to reinforce the notion that the perception of the world is never final.[3]

A famous Mazatec Shaman, Maria Sabina, described how she owed her insight to the plant world:

There is a world beyond ours, a world that is far away, nearby and invisible. And that is where God lives, where the dead live, the spirits and the saints, a world where everything has already happened and everything is known ... The sacred mushroom takes me by the hand and brings me to the world where everything is known. It is they, the sacred mushrooms, that speak in a way I understand. I ask them and they answer me. When I return ... I tell what they have told me and what they have shown me.[4]

All this, of course, may be seen merely as an interesting aside and little to do with the practical world of the twentieth-century herbalist. But the medicine and ways of the Shaman have important implications for us, for they ask that we look at plants not just as chemical entities but as purveyors of subtle energies that are the essence of life itself. They also demand that we recognize our absolute reliance on the plant kingdom, and on the earth herself. When native herb-doctors gather plants they invariably take care to first ask the plant for permission to take it from its mother, the earth. This is not superstition but a timely recognition of the debt that is owed to nature.

Modern science now agrees that humans and plants have a close ecological relationship, but these ties may go much further than the obvious food chain, which, through the nourishment of plants, ensures that a single cell or zygote can grow into a fully grown human being in about twenty years. It also goes beyond the other crucial dependency we have on plants: our breathing in the oxygen that plants, by photosynthesis, breathe out. A further debt to the plant world can be discovered in what some call a plant mystery.

We know what purpose most plant constituents serve. Ninety per cent of the weight of a plant is cellulose and water, which together provide a vegetable skeleton to support the plant, and a medium in which nutrients are dissolved and transported around it. Carbohydrates, like starches and sugars, together with oils, proteins, mineral salts and pigments, account for practically all the rest of the plant. But some plants produce so-called secondary plant products, such as the alkaloids nicotine, caffeine and morphine, which have marked physiological and psychic effects on human beings, yet have no apparent role in the plants themselves. Biologists have advanced several theories to try and explain the part these substances play in the life of a plant but none, on analysis, are really credible. For example, the explanation that these psychoactive compounds act as plant defence-mechanisms, preventing depredation by animals and insects, is hardly convincing, since most poisonous plants are in fact eaten by animals. There exists a beetle which lives exclusively on the leaves of deadly nightshade, and goats happily munch hemlock, which killed Socrates. Schultes and Hoffman observed, in their book *Plants of the Gods*: 'It remains . . . one of the unsolved riddles of nature why certain plants produce substances with specific effect on the mental and emotional function of man, on his sense of perception and actually on his state of consciousness.'[5]

However if we recognize the implications of the mutual relationship and interdependency of the plant and human realms, this is a riddle no longer. Plants possess, alongside their nutritive properties, other properties which can be physically healing and spiritually enhancing for human beings. In short, this is no coincidence. Herbalist David Hoffman argues that such thinking is in line with the Gaia hypothesis, proposed by former NASA scientist Jim Lovelock.[6] Gaia is the ancient Greek goddess of the earth, but Lovelock has further defined Gaia as a 'complex entity involving the earth's biosphere, oceans and soil, the totality constituting a feedback or cybernetic system, which seeks an optimal physical or chemical environment for life on this planet. The maintenance of relatively constant conditions by active control may be conveniently described as homeostasis.'[7] 'To what extent,' Lovelock asks, 'is our collective intelligence also a part of Gaia? Do we, as a species, constitute a Gaian nervous system?'

Whatever the answer, the idea of plants and man coexisting to support one another and the earth herself seems eminently reasonable to the herbalist. Intuitive herbal medicine may then be a direct connection with a collective

Gaian unconsciousness, which we do not explore enough in this formidably scientific age.

In time, a second method of herbal medicine displaced that of the Shaman. This change is often characterized as an escape from myth and magic into a more rational and logical system of medicine. Whether this is actually so or not, the change was brought about in ancient Greece by Hippocrates (who lived around 460–360 BC). Hippocrates declared that he was banishing superstition and magic from medicine. A skilled herbalist, he substituted a humoral or elemental system of evaluating his plant medicines and his patients for the direct intuition of the Shaman. (Although elemental medicine was common to Shamanism, it was perceived intuitively rather than intellectually.) We may call this later system both intuitive and logical. It is worth noting in passing that Hippocrates is known as the father of medicine, and that his approach emphasized the left-brained, more masculine and logical approach rather than the right-brained, feminine and intuitive herbalism of the Shaman. Ever since Hippocrates, medicine has become ever more objective and logical, with less room for subjective intuition. Perhaps it is no coincidence that it has become more male dominated too.*

As in Greece, the humoral system of herbal medicine replaced that of the Shaman in all other ancient cultures. Although these systems vary one from another in detail, a comparison shows certain common fundamental principles in action.

Hippocrates wrote:

The human body contains blood, phlegm, yellow bile and black bile. A man enjoys the most perfect health when these elements are duly proportioned to one another in power, bulk and manner

---

* See Oliver Sacks's fascinating book, *The Man who Mistook his Wife for a Hat*,[8] concerning neurology's left-brain bias: 'Indeed the entire history of neurology and neuropsychology can be seen as a history of the investigation of the left hemisphere.'

of compounding so that they are mingled as excellently as possible. Pain is felt when one of these elements is deficient or excessive or when it is isolated in the body without being compounded with the others.[9]

Such a view of health and disease emphasizes aspects of treatment quite alien to modern medicine. But its sentiments are echoed by most traditional systems of herbal medicine, and are still applicable today. The approaches of traditional herbalism and modern medicine are in stark contrast.

Fundamental to the herbal view is the concept that plants are used to restore *balance* and *harmony* to the patient. As Hippocrates indicates, disease is seen as a disharmony of the matter and energy that go to make up the human being (the word 'dis-ease' itself implies this). Plant medicines, so often akin to foods, are ideally suited to the role of restoring equilibrium. The surgical techniques and drugs of modern medicine, on the other hand, are aggressive measures to attack or contain disease, which is focused on as a clearly defined entity, often at the expense of the patient as a whole.

Modern medicine is dualistic because it is heir to the ideas of Descartes, who said that man consisted of two distinct parts – mind (*res cogitans*) and body (*res extensa*) – and that the body was merely a machine and disease a breakdown of the body's mechanism.

I wish you to consider, finally, that all the functions which I attribute to this machine, such as digestion ... nutrition ... respiration, waking and sleeping; the reception of light, sound, odours ... the impression of ideas on the memory; the inferior movements of the appetites and passions, and finally the movements of all the external members ... I desire ... that you consider these functions occur naturally in this machine, solely by the disposition of its organs, not less than the movements of a clock.[10]

Once the separation of mind and body was accepted, anatomical dissection was no longer reprehensible to the Church or State, and the way was open, via the scalpel of the anatomists, for disease to be defined, wherever possible, by what damage it did to healthy tissue (pathology).

Modern medicine, it follows then, is also reductionist, believing that everything that occurs in the human body – mental and emotional experiences included – may be completely explained in biochemical and bioelectrical terms. This outlook is in marked contrast to the perspective of the herbalist. Herbal traditions emphasize the indivisibility and interaction of mind and body, matter and spirit (see Appendix A). Hippocrates, for example, did not see his humours as mere physical characteristics, for they coloured all aspects of being – physical, mental and emotional. We recognize this today when we describe someone as having a phlegmatic temperament.

The humours and elements of traditional medical systems are the primordial description of all phenomena, animate and inanimate. And through all such phenomena, flowing like a tide, is the universal force or energy, recognized variously, with subtle differences of interpretation, from culture to culture. It is called *pneuma* by the Greeks, *prana* by the Indians, *Qi* by the Chinese and re-defined as the *vis medicatrix naturae*, or vital force, of modern times. But to the herbalist, regardless of training or tradition, the essential aim is the same: to provide the patient with herbs that can re-establish or revive the harmonious flow of this universal life force, without which we die and which itself is the true healer.

The next chapter details the way in which herbs are used to treat illness. But here suffice it to say that in contrast to the reductionist and analytical techniques of the orthodox doctor, the aim of the traditional herbalist is to piece together all the symptoms and signs and so obtain an overall view or pattern of the patient's disharmony, from which a herbal prescription can logically follow. In both eastern and western systems of traditional herbal medicine, practitioners construct an individual clinical picture by observing and questioning each patient about pain, temperature (hot or cold), appearance, skin function (e.g. sweating), appetite, thirst, urination and bowel movements.

The restoration of harmony is integral to Chinese herbal medicine. Harmonious balance is expressed in terms of the two complementary forces – yin and yang; and the five elements or phases – fire, earth, metal, water and wood. Wang Chhung, the great philosopher of the Han dynasty, explained how the harmonious interplay between yin and yang gives rise to life:

That by which man is born, are of the two Qi of the Yin and Yang. The Yin Qi produces his bones and flesh; the Yang Qi his vital spirit. As long as he is alive, the Yin and Yang are in good order, hence the bones and flesh are strong and the vital force full of vigour.[11]

The five elements are of particular importance to the Chinese herbalist; they give rise to the five tastes by which all medicinal plants are evaluated. In this way fire gives rise to bitterness, earth to sweetness, metal to acridity, water to saltiness and wood to sourness. Each taste is said to have a particular medicinal action: bitter-tasting herbs drain and dry; sweet herbs tonify and may reduce pain; acrid herbs disperse; salty herbs nourish the kidneys; while sour herbs nourish the yin and astringe, preventing unwanted loss of body fluids or Qi. Herbs which have none of these tastes are described as bland – a taste which indicates that the plant may have a diuretic effect. The taste of a plant can also indicate the organ to which it has natural affinity. So the Yellow Emperor's *Classic of Internal Medicine* states that 'Sourness enters the liver, acridity the lungs, bitterness the heart, saltiness the kidneys and sweetness the spleen'.[12]

Besides defining particular herbal tastes, the Chinese, in common with herbalists from other cultures, ascribe different temperatures to herbs. These are, again, five in number: hot, cold, warm, cool and neutral. For instance, prepared aconite is one of the hottest herbs in the Chinese materia medica, while rhubarb root is one of the coldest. Traditional Chinese herbalists using this knowledge still follow the advice of the Yellow Emperor's *Classic of Internal Medicine*: 'Hot diseases must be cooled, cold diseases must be warmed', a piece of advice echoed by Paracelsus when, many centuries later, he wrote, 'Every remedy given should be taken from precisely that force in Nature which is brother to the failing force within the human body; by such means are the macrocosmic forces renewed within the microscopic man.'[13]

The subjective temperatures and tastes of plants were of equal interest to ancient Greek and Indian herbalists. Aristotle emphasized the dynamic nature of the four Greek elements – earth, air, fire and water – by considering the qualities of cold, dry, hot and moist. Throughout the Middle Ages, this energetic description was applied to herbs (just as the *Classic of Internal Medicine* also advised) to indicate how they could be used. John Gerard, herbalist to James I, is recorded as describing 'aconite and garlic as hot and dry in the fourth degree', and explaining that garlic 'is an enemie to all cold poisons'. In 1957 a scientific report showed that garlic indeed contains a powerful antibacterial agent, allicin, so backing up Gerard's claim.

The Ayurvedic or ancient Indian system of medicine also recognized five elements: aether, fire, water, air and earth. These five elements manifest themselves in the body to form the *Tridosha*, or three basic humours: *vata* (the principle of air or movement); *pitta* (the principle of fire); and *kapha* (the principle of water). Like the Greek and Chinese medical systems, Ayurvedic medicine perceived all universal energies as having their counterparts within the human being, and so the healing process sought to achieve, in individuals, a balance between the elements of air or wind (*vata*), fire or bile (*pitta*), and water or phlegm (*kapha*). Ayurvedic medicine likewise insisted that the taste of a herb is not incidental, but is indicative of its properties. The Sanskrit word for taste, *rasa*, means 'essence'. In the Ayurvedic system there are six essences: sweet, sour, salty, pungent, bitter and astringent. As in Chinese herbal medicine, the Ayurvedic herbals categorized all plants according to this system, so that their herbalists could make out prescriptions more easily. For example, Ayurveda taught that pungent, sour and salty-tasting herbs cause heat, and so increase *pitta* (fire); sweet, bitter and astringent herbs had precisely an opposite effect, cooling and decreasing *pitta*.

Tibetan herbal medicine, like that of India, seeks balance between three humours – bile, wind and phlegm. Once again each herb is categorized according to its taste, and also according to its relationship to the three elements. The Tibetans recognize six tastes: sweet, sour, bitter, astringent, hot and salty. They believe the universe to be composed of five constituents: earth, water, fire, air and space. Bile has the nature of fire; phlegm the nature of earth; water and wind the nature of movement.

It is fascinating to see that these concepts – that is, the need to restore harmony and re-balance to the body's systems by using herbs, which aid the vital force – are similarly at the heart of a system of medicine that flourished at the end of the nineteenth century in the USA. This was the physiomedical system of herbal medicine, which, as we have seen, was founded by Samuel Thomson (1769–1843), who drew on the herbal skills of the North American Indians and herb lore imported to America by the early European settlers. Physiomedicalism was eventually legislated out of existence in America, but it still has great influence amongst present-day herbal practitioners in the UK.

Thomson's theories in many respects resembled, and yet were years in advance of, the later German pioneers of 'nature cure' (naturopathy). The reason for this is that Thomson insisted on the predominance of the vital force which he defined as that directive intelligence in us all, always seeking to resist inimical outside influences – whether bacterial, viral or climatic – and always seeking to restore health by eliminating accumulated toxins (a phenomenon called homoeostasis by modern science).

There are also striking parallels between Thomson's ideas and those expressed in one of the most famous of all Chinese herbals – the *Shang-han Lun* (*Discussion of Cold-induced Disorders*) – written around AD 220 by Zhang Zhong-jing, a man nicknamed 'the Chinese Hippocrates'. Thomson held that all bodies were composed of the four elements – earth, air, fire and water – and health derived from their harmonious interplay. He saw cold, or a reduction of heat, as a major cause of disease, and so recommended methods to restore this imbalance using steam baths and hot, stimulating herbs like cayenne pepper. Zhang Zhong-jing was, likewise, mainly concerned with disease brought on by cold. The most frequently prescribed herb in the *Shang-han Lun* is cinnamon, which, like cayenne pepper, has stimulating, warming and diaphoretic properties. Both men worked during times when ordinary people lived a rugged, tough, outdoor life; malnutrition, hypothermia and exhaustion were major causes of illness. As a result the essential thrust of their herbal therapies was to stimulate and warm their patients, whose body-resistance was severely reduced.

Thomson's vigorous methods of treatment, which included liberal doses of emetic herbs like lobelia, were appropriate for his time but required refinement to meet the changing needs of future generations. One can clearly see how the character of herbal treatment employed by the developing physiomedical school evolved to meet problems thrown up by different living conditions. Dr Wooster Beach, who published his *American Practice* in 1842, criticized Thomson for using too much cayenne pepper, arguing that hot *or* cold could precipitate disease. In hot diseases he advised the use of cold or tepid bathing, together with strong infusions of catnep, to eliminate toxins by sweating. In China a more gradual evolution, following the same pattern, occurred, marked by the 1746 publication of Dr Ye Tian Shi's *Wen Bing Lun (Treatise on Warm Diseases)*. Later, the English herbalist John Skelton writing around 1870, when his herbal surgery was filled with men, women and children suffering diseases directly attributable to the appalling pollution and hardship of the Industrial Revolution, emphasized the need to purify the patient's blood because of the 'constant deterioration of the blood from impure air and exhaustion by day, bad ventilation at night, and want of attention to the ordinary requirements of life'.[14] Skelton used many blood-purifying herbs like nettles, burdock, yellow dock, red clover and cleavers.

Life-styles continued to change and physiomedical practitioners like J. M. Thurston, who practised at the turn of the century, prophetically paid more attention to supporting and re-balancing the nervous system. Today, when such a large percentage of the patients visiting our herbal clinics have obvious nervous problems and neuroses caused by the intense pace and stress of twentieth-century life, we follow Thurston's example.

Thurston displayed the physiomedicalist's ability to synthesize the old and new. For example, to help determine his diagnosis and treatment he categorized his patients according to the traditional humoral or constitutional types – sanguine, bilious (or choleric), phlegmatic and melancholic (or nervous). On the other hand, the latest physiological discoveries of his time influenced the way he designed herbal prescriptions, for much of his work was aimed at balancing out the autonomic nervous system. Like all physiomedicalists, he relied on a simple but effective therapeutic formula to achieve this, which was *relax, astringe* and *stimulate*. W. H. Cook, a predecessor of Thurston, explained the rationale of this strategy:

Regularity in periods of alternate labour and rest is characteristic of all vital action . . . The duration of an effort in any organ may have considerable range, but relaxation must come, or the part will suffer from not receiving (in rest) a supply of nutrient equal to its waste . . . The earliest departure of the tissues from under the full control of the vital force will be in lack of ability either to relax or contract some of the tissues as readily as in the healthy state. The balance of complementary action is lost; and either the tendency to contractility increases while the power of relaxation diminishes, or laxity of the structures becomes more marked as the power to affect their contraction gets less . . . This loss of equilibrium constitutes a primary element in most diseases.[15]

The physiomedicalists used stimulating herbs like cayenne or ginger to revive deficient function, relaxant herbs like lobelia, wild yam and cramp bark to ease over-contracted tissues, and astringent herbs like geranium and bayberry to contract over-relaxed states.* They made full

* To the original formula, *relax, astringe* and *stimulate*, a fourth vector, *sedate*, was sometimes added. But many physiomedicalists preferred to avoid strongly sedative herbs which were often poisonous (e.g. opium), because they believed that one could not have too much vital force, and it was only necessary to *relax* the tissues to allow the body's energy to flow smoothly.

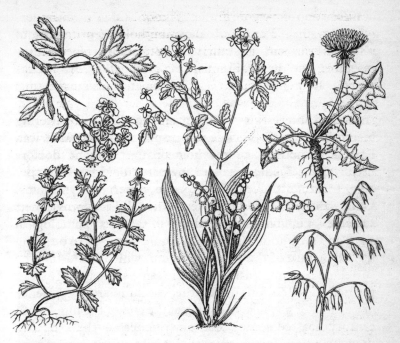

Hawthorn, Greater celandine, Dandelion, Eyebright, Lily of the valley, Wild oat

use of the empirical know-how of traditional herbalism, which held that particular herbs have specific actions. Experience proved that herbs could be diuretic (increasing the flow of urine), diaphoretic (increasing sweating), laxative, antispasmodic, carminative, expectorant, emmenagogic (bringing on menstruation), anthelmintic (expelling worms), and so on. In addition, some herbs have an affinity for particular organs or tissues. Eyebright, as the name suggests, is for eye problems (it is also astringent), lily of the valley and hawthorn are for the heart and circulation, dandelion root for the liver, greater celandine for the gall bladder, wild oats for the nervous system, cornsilk for the kidneys; the list continues. Although there has been

a huge leap forward in terms of physiological understanding since Thurston's day, the holistic principles of
physiomedicalism are still valid. In many respects they
resemble the basic premise of osteopathy and chiro-
practic, both developed at approximately the same time
in the USA.

A third interesting variation on the theme of differing
methods of herbal practice was displayed by the American
Eclectic School. Like the homeopaths, Eclectic doctors
used single remedies, prescribing particular plants for specific treatments according to the observed symptoms.
Unlike the homeopaths however they did not prove their
remedies, i.e. give material doses to see what pathological
signs and symptoms the remedy would provoke, so building
up the picture of that very symptom, which could then be
corrected by a minimal dose of the same substance. Instead
the Eclectics drew on the recorded, accumulated experience
of a school of physicians, which at the end of the nineteenth
century boasted some 8,000 practitioners in the USA, to
draw up a symptom-picture that would clearly indicate the
specific use of any remedy. One of the most famous Eclectic
practitioners, John Scudder (1829–94), argued that herbal
compounds and mixtures should be abandoned, and in their
place he proposed that physicians should study and prescribe according to 'the direct action of single drugs'. Such
an approach required detailed knowledge of the specific
effect of each remedy on the body. Writing in his famous
Eclectic Materia Medica: Pharmacology and Therapeutics,
published in 1922, Harvey Wicks Felter, a professor at the
Eclectic Medical College of Cincinnati, summed up the
Eclectic endeavour:

Conservatism and fidelity to the experiences of the many, rather
than the record of the merely new, novel or bizarre, and gener-
alizations rather than the single experience in drug therapy, have
been kept uppermost . . . and wherever possible the specific use

of specific means, according to established specific indications, has been given preference to other forms of medication.

We have now discussed three of the four main ways of working with herbs and so come to the fourth, which is that of modern scientific herbalism.

In the last hundred years or so plant chemists have demonstrated that many traditional herbal remedies contain chemical constituents which have a measurable activity in the body, and which correspond to the way the whole plant was traditionally used. Some herbalists prescribe plants more or less entirely according to their known pharmacological constituents to treat specific diseases. This is done without any reference to the traditional properties of the plant, such as its tendency to heat or cool, stimulate or relax. Such an approach, in my opinion, is not holistic herbalism in its true sense, but advocates of this method correctly argue that the whole plant acts much more gently within the body than the isolated, active chemical constituents, and so is preferable to orthodox drug therapy.

Science and folklore have recently worked together to rediscover the medicinal properties of the plant feverfew, which has been hailed as a specific for migraines. Attention first focused on feverfew when the wife of the chief medical officer for the National Coal Board was given a cutting of the plant by a miner, with which to treat her headaches. After eating a leaf or two every day for fourteen months, her headaches ceased. Medical researchers became interested, and in a preliminary trial on migraine sufferers seven out of ten patients claimed that their migraine attacks were less frequent, less painful, or both. About a third of the patients treated reported that they suffered no further migraine attacks at all.[16] It is interesting that John Parkinson (whom we met in Chapter 1) wrote of this herb, 'It is very effectual for all paines in the head, coming of a cold cause, as Camerius saith, the hearbe being bruised and applied to crowne of the head.'[17] In 1772 John Hill wrote, 'In the worst headache this herb exceeds whatever else is known.'[18]

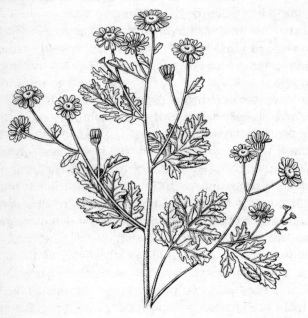

Feverfew

In France, for the treatment of infectious disease, some doctors have now substituted antibiotics with volatile oils. Dr Paul Belaiche, who holds the newly created chair of herbal medicine at the University of Paris North, has, using a volatile oil technique, achieved a success rate of more than eighty per cent in his treatment of several thousand women suffering from intractable cystitis. Again, it seems to me that this is not holistic herbalism, but it is not drug therapy either, for volatile oils used in tiny amounts do no damage to the body when they kill off bacteria. On the other hand, this kind of treatment does tend to lose sight of the overall view of the patient.

Today herbal students study the chemistry of plants, for it is rightly recognized that such study enhances the skill of the herbal practitioner. We look at some plant chemical components in Chapter 6. As we have seen, an enormous number of modern drugs have been derived from herbal medicines. But herbal practitioners profoundly disagree with isolating and synthesizing the active principles of herbs to use as drugs. These isolated chemicals, taken out of context, are, in the long term, often incompatible with good health. The experience of the herbalist is that the whole plant is greater than the sum of its constituent parts, and that the multiplicity of chemical components, most of which – although apparently pharmacologically inert – can play a significant role in the body. They either make the recognized active constituents biologically available, or buffer the powerful action of potent plant chemicals, so preventing possible harmful side-effects. A few specific examples help to illustrate this important point.

Digitalis v. digoxin

Dr William Thomson, former editor of *Black's Medical Dictionary*, cites digoxin as an example of how drug companies have been rash to assume an isolated plant chemical is better medicine than the whole herb.

Although you could overdose from taking the digitalis leaf, this did not happen with anything like the regularity we experienced with the isolated glycosides. The drug companies found a market largely because digitalis preparations, especially the tinctures, got a name for unreliability. This was simply due to the fact that chemists tended to keep them on their shelves too long, until they had lost much of their power.[19]

Dr Thomson goes on to say:

There is no convincing evidence that any of the individual glycosides in use today have any advantage over digitalis leaf . . . and
it is not irrelevant to note a recent report showing that one in
four patients with heart conditions treated by the most widely
used of these digitalis glycosides was found to be suffering from
an overdose of the drug, and that of these patients, one in sixteen
died of digitalis poisoning.[20]

Ephedra sinica v. ephedrine

The Chinese herb ma huang is the source of the alkaloid
ephedrine, which was extracted from *Ephedra sinica* by
Japanese scientists in 1885. It was hailed as a potent
bronchodilator – relaxing the airways of the respiratory
system – and so was recognized to be of particular use in
treating asthmatics. Unfortunately, once in widespread use,
the isolated drug was found markedly to raise blood pressure, and so now it is hardly ever used to treat asthma. But
contained in the whole plant are six other related alkaloids,
one of them being pseudo-ephedrine, which actually
reduces the heart rate and lowers the blood pressure. This
plant has been used in China for thousands of years and no
undesirable side-effects have been recorded as a result of
the proper administration of the whole plant.

Rauwolfia serpentina v. reserpine

Rauwolfia was first mentioned in the *Charka Samhita*, an
Ayurvedic medical treatise dating from around 1000 BC. In
1952 an alkaloid called reserpine was extracted from the
plant. A few grams of this white crystalline substance were

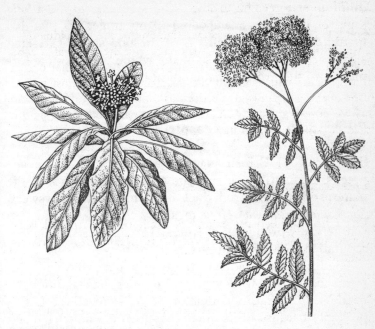

Rauwolfia, Meadowsweet

as potent as more than 10,000 times the weight of the root itself. Reserpine was hailed as a wonder-drug for the treatment of high blood pressure, but it was not long before alarming reports were coming in from doctors who had been prescribing it for hypertension. Apparently this new drug was throwing patients who had been mentally stable into acute manic-depressive states. Today reserpine is a more or less forgotten drug, abandoned due to its alarming side-effects. Yet a tea made of an infusion of the whole plant had, for many centuries, been a famous Indian folk-remedy for madness and hysteria. It gained its Hindi name, *Chandra*, meaning moon, because of its calming effect on lunacy. This tea was traditionally given to fretful Indian babies, and Mahatma Gandhi regularly drank it for its calming effect. The whole plant contains at least one hundred and sixty-one alkaloids;[21] the tragedy is that due to the disastrous side-effects of the one single extracted alkaloid, reserpine, the use of the whole plant is now forbidden to the professional medical herbalist.

Filipendula ulmaria *v.* aspirin

The beautiful British plant meadowsweet contains appreciable quantities of salicylic acid (aspirin). Indeed the name aspirin comes from the Latin name for meadowsweet, *Spirea ulmaria* – *a spirea* meaning without the aid (i.e. synthetically produced) of spirea. The plant has an ancient reputation for treating arthritic pain. As aspirin, the isolated salicylic acid has frequently been the cause of stomach ulcers. Meadowsweet, however, has traditionally been used to treat inflammation of the stomach (gastritis), probably because of its other constituents – mucilage and tannin – which tend to protect the stomach lining from the corrosive effect of the salicylates it contains.

CHAPTER THREE

PRACTICE

Let us now have a look at the ideas discussed in Chapter 2 when they are put into practice. Here we consider how herbs are used to treat both acute and chronic disease. Since my training is in both the eastern and western traditions, and both are currently available in this country, it also seems relevant to make comparisons, and draw parallels, between these two approaches to specific problems. In so doing, it will become increasingly apparent that there are many similarities between the different herbal systems, whose origins are separated by thousands of miles and years. Insight, of course, is not the prerogative of any one culture or time. Such similarities are enlightening, but not surprising.

We begin by considering the treatment of fever, which usually develops quite suddenly and is associated with rapid physiological changes that tend to last a relatively short time – all features characteristic of acute disease. Fevers, of course, can also be chronic (chronic disease has a relatively long duration), but that is another subject.

Allopathic medicine usually directly opposes fever through the administration of antipyretic drugs, such as aspirin, which lower the temperature by acting on the hypothalamus – the heat-regulating centre, similar to a thermostat, situated in the brain. Antibiotics are also often prescribed, their purpose being to destroy the infecting bacteria seen to cause the fever. Fever is of course just a symptom of a greater malady. Suppressing it by such measures begs two pertinent questions. First, what is the purpose of fever itself, and second, why does it so often happen that one person succumbs to infection, while those around him or her remain immune?

Modern physiology answers the first question, recognizing, at least in theory, the value of fever. A standard textbook of pharmacology observes: 'An increased temperature may not only increase the reactions of the body to infection, but may also directly injure the organisms causing infection.'[1] The knowledge that infecting organisms die at higher than normal body temperatures was the basis of a heroic treatment for syphilis of the central nervous system, which was controlled by deliberately infecting the patient with malaria, so causing regular bouts of high fever. Once the syphilis had been burnt out, the malaria was then treated.

The same pharmacology textbook continues: 'Reducing the temperature of a fevered patient generally makes him more comfortable, but may delay his cure and cause his collapse.' But this caution is usually ignored both by doctors and patients, who tend to use antipyretic drugs as soon as fever occurs.

A moment of reflection will reveal an obvious illogicality here. If fever itself is antibiotic, it makes no sense to suppress it while at the same time taking antibiotics. Surely no one questions the value of drugs like antibiotics *in extremis*, but each and every one of us experiences febrile episodes, which are not life-threatening and do not deserve to be managed in this way.* This is certainly the view of the herbalist, who sees fever as a positive and reconstructive effort by the vital force of the body to eliminate toxins. Herbal medicines are prescribed to facili-

---

* Such measures may be unsafe for other reasons too. Aspirin, the most commonly used of these drugs, was first introduced into medicine in 1899 and has, since June 1986, been prohibited for treating children under twelve, since it has been linked to the incidence of Raye's syndrome, which causes brain and kidney damage in the young.

tate this essentially healthy process which should not be suppressed.

The question of why one person gets an infection while others in close contact with the sick person do not, is also answered by the herbalist. Bacteria and viruses are recognized as merely precipitating or exciting causes of disease, but the underlying cause is the state of lowered resistance or vitality of the sick person. Although many herbs have a scientifically demonstrable antibiotic action, a fever calls for an assessment of the patient's own vital energy and medicines to support this, rather than only using herbs which wage war on the infecting organism. Tonification is a notion quite foreign to modern medicine, but herbs which supply trace elements, vitamins and gentle stimulation, while encouraging the elimination of waste materials and toxins, certainly justify their tonic reputation. They are ideal agents to help recovery from the long-term sequelae of a debilitating disease, like glandular fever (mononucleosis), where modern medicine has nothing much to offer.

I have often found, when talking to doctors about herbal medicine, that they react with frank incredulity whenever I mention the idea of herbal tonics. But the notion of tonic herbs has received some support in a recent *Guardian* article:

Non-western systems of medicine . . . do not deal primarily in physic but in tonics. In mainland Europe too, this ancient system of tonics persists, witness the herbalists of France. But we, I'm sure, are missing out, more grouchy, more tired, perhaps more susceptible to infection or maybe chronic disease, because our metabolism is deprived of a thousand subtle lubricants to which it is pre-adapted. Perhaps in a few decades or so . . . nutritionalists and pharmacologists . . . will turn their attention to what are considered to be the fringes, beginning with the nostrums of the herbalist and apothecaries and make them scientifically respectable. Then perhaps we'll allow ourselves to espouse the primitive diet in all its glory.[2]

When it comes to treating fever, as in the approach to other illnesses, both eastern and western systems of herbal medicine stress treatment of the patient and not the disease. The physiomedical herbalists in America, who laid down methods of practice now followed by many herbalists in the UK, broadly differentiated between two kinds of acute fever, based on the fundamental strength or weakness of a patient. This idea follows logically from the notion that acute fever is a healthy reaction to toxic invasion. Thus the stronger and more healthy the patient, the more marked the fever, while patients in whom the vital force is weak will experience an incompetent type of fever. About the former kind of fever, W. H. Cook, the physiomedical herbalist, wrote:

The shiverings and rigors of the onset are distinct; the febrile reaction is prompt and strong with a rather high temperature. Pains in the limbs and headache are marked, headache is frequently throbbing; the pulse is large, firm and strong; the skin is very hot and dry; digestion is disturbed, with a thickly furred and moist tongue, disagreeable thirst and constipation . . . such a grade of fever indicates great vital strength.[3]

Of the weaker type of fever he wrote:

The vital vigour is much reduced; the weakness and sense of prostration are marked, and febrile action is feeble. The pulse is small, rapid and weak; the tongue continues moist and is usually pale and flabby.* The thirst is moderate . . . it is one of the low types of fevers, and not favourable.[4]

* Here is a good example of parallel practice in eastern and western herbalism. Pulse and tongue diagnosis, usually associated with Indian, Chinese and Tibetan medicine, is also important to western herbalists in the physiomedical tradition. Western physiomedicalist Dr Lyle wrote: 'Each disease makes itself felt on the circulation. This is why we feel a pulse to discern its character and the degree of vital resistance . . . The pulse and tongue are the two great indexes to the abnormal conditions of the body. The former indicates the degree that the abnormal condition is felt by the circulation, and the latter the degree that is felt by the digestive organs.'[5]

The two contrasting pictures of fever are treated quite differently. The full fever calls for herbs which are *relaxing* and make the patient sweat (diaphoretic). Such sweating goes beyond just cooling out the fever; it also eliminates wastes and toxins. In this kind of fever it is quite unnecessary to use stimulants like cayenne (*capsicum minimum*), since there is plenty of inner vitality. Here herbs are selected to encourage a free outward flow of energy, which if blocked will lead to inner congestion and complications. The repression of fevers with drugs is often responsible for subsequent chronic disease. It is even possible mistakenly to suppress a moderate fever by using cold ice packs or water, so that the fever cannot do its work.

In the case of strong fever the herbalist might use the following prescription:

Equal parts of:
Elderflower (*Sambucus nigra*)
Catnep (*Nepeta cataria*)
Pleurisy root (*Asclepias tuberosa*)

All three of these herbs have a gentle relaxing effect on the skin and capillaries, promoting a good, free sweat. A hot infusion is the preferred method of administration to treat this condition, because its heat encourages the diaphoretic action of the herbs. Starving a fever is also a good idea; it leaves the body free to fight off the infection. Of course most people with fever lose their appetites anyway.

In contrast, when the fever is weak, the herbalist needs to prescribe gentle herbal *stimulants*, and *stimulating* diaphoretic herbs, to support the ailing vital force and bring about a therapeutic sweat. Here the stimulating diaphoretics are ginger or wild ginger (*Asarum canadense*) in a hot infusion together with yarrow (*Achillea millefolium*) and boneset (*Eupatorium perfoliatum*). Prickly ash (*Xanthoxylum americanum*) or bayberry (*Myrica cerifera*) can be added as stimulants. The astringent action of bayberry contracts and tones the arteries, improving blood flow outwards.

The physiomedical herbalists saw four distinct stages in a typical acute fever: a premonitory period when the patient probably felt a little off-colour; a cold stage, as the fever rose, when the patient felt cold and shivery; a hot stage, as the fever reached its zenith; and finally, if all went well, a return to norm. Bearing in mind that it is easier to coax the vital force than to drive it, herbalists tailor their prescriptions to fit this natural cycle. For instance, the cold stage might be treated by hot water baths, containing infusions of warming and stimulating herbs like ginger and cinnamon, or a little oil of rosemary. Similarly, warming herbs like prickly ash (*Xanthoxylum americanum*) or ginger, which encourage blood flow outwards, to warm cold extremities, can also be taken internally. To these may be added antibiotic herbs like echinacea (*Echinacea angustifolia*), or wild indigo (*Baptisia tinctoria*).*

Chinese herbalists also see fever as occurring in stages. Two famous schemes map out these stages, from which the herbalist can work out his or her treatment. One from the *Shang-han Lun* (*Discussion of Cold-induced Disorders*) is in six stages and begins with fever induced by cold or chills, while the other, devised during the Ming and Qing dynasties, proposes a four-stage cycle similar to the western scheme. In the case of the four-stage cycle, the cause of fever is heat rather than cold. The second stage of both these schemes describes a high fever with marked sweating, a great thirst, and a rapid, bounding pulse. Here the Chinese-style herbalist might use a famous prescription

---

* It seems that herbal antibiotics, like echinacea, work by stimulating the body's own defences, for example increasing production of white blood cells, which attack invading bacteria.

which also dates back to the *Shang-han Lun* called White Tiger Soup (*Bai Hu Tang*). There are no bits of tiger in this prescription. It gets this name because traditionally tigers were seen by the Chinese to be yin and white tigers even more so. Here a cooling, yin-tonifying mixture of herbs moistens and soothes the yang excesses of a full-fire high fever (see Appendix B).

Like their western counterparts, Chinese herbalists view acute fever as a healthy reaction to a pathogenic factor. Its immediate cause is usually seen as an attack by hostile, exterior climatic conditions (so-called 'evils'), mostly either wind and cold or wind and heat. These 'evils' battle with the body's first line of defence – the defensive Qi or energy (*Wei Qi*) – which flows between the skin and muscles. The stronger the defensive Qi, and the more virulent the invading 'evil', the more fiercely burns the fever. A low or chronic fever is therefore a sign of a weak constitution since it implies weak Qi.

If a person's lifestyle and rising and retiring are abnormal, or cold and warmth are not adjusted, or there is exhaustion from overwork, the subcutaneous space becomes slack and *Wei Qi* ceases to be firm and there is great susceptibility to occupation by external evils.

Nei-Ke-Xue, *a modern textbook on traditional Chinese medicine.*[6]

The traditional Chinese physician distinguishes, by pulse and tongue, the signs and symptoms of the fever, whether the offending 'evil' is wind-cold or wind-heat (or perhaps some other far less common factor). For example, fever accompanied by copious sweating is an important clue, indicating wind-heat 'evil'. Conversely, lack of sweating in someone with fever may indicate attack by wind-cold. If the fevered patient is thirsty, this indicates heat, while a patient with a raised temperature who is not very thirsty may well have a wind-cold condition.

Once the diagnosis is made, a traditional prescription is selected to restore balance in the body. A commonly used prescription for wind-cold affliction has the rather fearsome name of the Schizonepeta-Ledebouriella Defeating Poisons Powder (*Jing-Fang Bai-Du San*) (see Appendix B). Although this is sold in Chinese pharmacies as a powder, it is better given as a hot decoction because the hot drink reinforces the main effect of the prescription, which is to provoke a sweat in order to disperse the wind-cold evil. This follows the ancient Chinese saying: 'When disease is in the skin, sweating will drive it out.' As we have seen, western herbalists would applaud this strategy.

Another famous prescription called, more poetically, Honeysuckle-Forsythia Powder (*Yin-Qiao San*) is used to counteract fever caused by wind-heat evil. In this case a powder is the normal way to give the remedy; the extra heat induced by drinking a hot decoction is seen to be counter-productive for this hot condition. The prescription of ten herbs (see Appendix B) may have herbs subtracted or added according to the patient's need. A frequent addition for instance is dyer's woad (*Isatis tinctoria*), which, like the honeysuckle and forsythia contained in the prescription, western research has shown to have definite antibiotic properties. Dyer's woad was traditionally used for epidemics of contagious diseases that afflicted people regardless of their constitutional strength. The overall effect of this powder is to cool and clear heat, and to disperse the exterior 'evil' by causing sweating.

To sum up, fevers are treated by western and Chinese-style herbalists in essentially the same way. Fever is never suppressed. Instead the patient's body is cooled or relaxed (or warmed or stimulated, if necessary), and cleansed by the use of herbs which encourage sweating. As the fever rises and falls, prescriptions are carefully chosen to suit the changing requirements of the patient.

Herbal remedies can be equally effective in reversing chronic disease, even after many years. Indeed the large majority of patients who consult herbalists today suffer from long-term, rather than acute, problems. Unfortunately, all too often the herbalist is the last resort and is only asked for help when the situation has become grave, or more or less irreversible. Nevertheless, even in these cases there is usually something that can be done.

The key to the herbal treatment of chronic disease is *slow and gently does it* (quite a contrast to modern drug therapy). Toxic elements, like tissue wastes or fatty deposits, accumulated over many years, may be gently released using deep acting depurative herbs. Western herbalists call depurative herbs 'alteratives'. They include burdock (*Arctium lappa*), figwort (*Scrophularia nodosa*), blue flag (*Iris versicolor*) and yellow dock (*Rumex crispus*). However, alteratives can begin working only after the organs and channels of elimination, particularly the kidneys and bowel, have been helped to function properly. For example, cornsilk (*Zea mays*) and goosegrass (*Galium aparine*) can be used to encourage this cleansing process, via the kidneys. To do otherwise may provoke a crisis, as the alterative herbs cause toxins to be released from the tissues, which then cannot be expelled by the body. For this reason, it is also important to ensure that the liver – the body's waste-material plant, excreting bile-pigments, urea and various detoxification products – is functioning properly. This is especially so today when so many patients visiting the herbalist have been taking highly potent and toxic drugs for many years. Liver remedies, such as dandelion root (*Taraxacum officinale*) and barberry bark (*Berberis vulgaris*), are frequently added to herbal prescriptions. The state of the circulation, the body's great highway, and its pump, the heart, also needs assessing.

Again the herbal pharmacopeia is replete with remedies to restore function, such as lily of the valley (*Convallaria majalis*) and hawthorn (*Crataegus oxyacanthoides*) for the heart; ginger, prickly ash (*Xanthoxylum americanum*) and bayberry bark (*Myrica cerifera*) for the arterial circulation; golden seal (*Hydrastis canadensis*) for the venous circulation, and so on.

It is important for the herbalist to pay attention to the energy reserves of the patient before setting about cleansing the system with alterative herbs. If the patient is weak, this cleansing process should be delayed until gentle, stimulating tonics have increased health and strength. This can be achieved by using gastro-intestinal tonics like gentian root (*Gentiana lutea*), and nervine tonics like skullcap (*Scutellaria lateriflora*) and wild oats (*Avena sativa*). In this way the western herbalist evaluates each of the body's systems in turn, providing stimulating or relaxing remedies as they are needed.

Finally, to illustrate the treatment of chronic disease, we briefly look at the case of three patients, both from the standpoint of the herbalist trained in the western way, and from that of a Chinese-style herbalist. The ingredients for these and all further treatments are given in metric quantities. There should, however, be no significant discrepancies if the following rounded equivalents are used:

Liquid weight	Dry weight
5 ml–1 tsp	2.5 gm–1 tsp
8 ml–$\frac{1}{4}$ fl oz	8 gm–$\frac{1}{4}$ oz
30 ml–1 fl oz	30 gm–1 oz
500 ml–1 pt	500 gm–1 lb
1 litre–2 pt	1 kg–2 lb

Case 1

Peter X; thirty-three years old; successful programmer for a big computer company. Happily married with two children. No health problems until a year previously when he began to suffer from a dull pain above the navel, usually shortly after eating. Pains are now more frequent (occurring several times a week) together with a loss of appetite, slight nausea and belching. He has experienced occasional diarrhoea recently. He visited his GP, and a gastro-enterologist, where he was given a barium meal and gastro-scopy, which revealed some inflammation of the stomach lining but no ulceration. The patient gained only slight relief from the drugs he was given. He says the pain is often worse after drinking coffee and eating bread and cheese. It is relieved by pressing his abdomen and warm drinks. Peter X works long hours, often skipping meals or eating late at night. His favourite meal is fish, chips and mushy peas. He does not drink much alcohol, or smoke. He has been feeling tired lately, and mentions that his grandfather died of a perforated ulcer.

Examination

The patient looked pale and drawn. Palpation of the abdomen revealed a tense, slightly painful area above the navel (epigastric area). Pulse: thin and soft. Tongue: pale with a white coat. All other examinations normal.

Western herbalist

ANALYSIS

Disturbance of the digestion and inflammation of the stomach lining. Digestive tract derangement can be gathered from the nausea, belching, loss of appetite and occasional diarrhoea; inflammation from the pain that occurs after meals and, of course, the result of the gastro-scopy.

The conclusion that the patient's vital energy is low can be deduced from his pale, drawn appearance, the chronic nature of the complaint, the soft, weak pulse, pale tongue, and the fact that he feels tired. Overlying the generally atonic or over-relaxed condition of the digestive system is local tension and over-contraction at the site of pain found at the physical examination.

PREDISPOSING CAUSES
Family history (grandfather's perforated ulcer); irregular eating; eating fried foods; coffee, bread and cheese; long hours of work: all have combined to bring about the present unhappy state of affairs.

STRATEGY
Relax, soothe and heal the stomach lining; tone the digestion by using astringent remedies and gastro-intestinal tonics. Support the nervous system.

PRESCRIPTION:
Tinctures of:
Comfrey (*Symphytum officinale*) 20 ml
Liquorice (*Glycyrrhiza glabra*) 7.5 ml
Golden seal (*Hydrastis canadensis*) 7.5 ml
Agrimony (*Agrimonia eupatoria*) 15 ml
Wild oats (*Avena sativa*) 10 ml
Chamomile (*Matricaria chamomilla*) 5 ml
Add water to 100 ml.

Take a teaspoon of tincture, diluted in warm water, after meals, three times daily. Once the pain and soreness have gone, the chamomile can be omitted and the prescription adjusted to include more stimulating and tonifying remedies such as gentian (*Gentiana lutea*), ginger and angelica (*Angelica archangelica*).

EXPLANATION OF THE PRESCRIPTION

Comfrey and **liquorice** both have a healing and soothing effect on the stomach lining. A study, undertaken in 1983 at King's College Hospital Medical School, showed that an aqueous extract of comfrey activated local hormones called prostaglandins, which can protect the stomach lining against inflammation. Comfrey also contains allantoin, which is a natural cell-healer. Liquorice, too, has been shown to have a marked action on the digestive system – relaxing spasms of the stomach and intestine, healing the inflamed stomach lining and lowering stomach-acid levels. **Golden seal** is a specific tonic and healing agent to the mucous membranes of the digestive tract. Its bitter taste stimulates the appetite. **Chamomile** is gently relaxing for the nervous system, helping also locally to relax spasms due to the damaged lining of the stomach. It also has an anti-inflammatory action. **Agrimony** gently stimulates and astringes the lining of the digestive tract. The astringent action tones and heals the damaged mucous membrane, and restores lower-bowel tone. This remedy encourages assimilation of foods, restoring a weakened digestion. **Wild oats** gently stimulate and nourish the nervous system.

Once the patient is no longer in pain, a further selection of herbs can be beneficially added to the prescription. These include **gentian**, a bitter tonic, stimulating peristaltic (wave-like) digestive activity, gastric secretions, the absorption of nutrients, and improving the appetite. **Angelica** is a warming and stimulating bitter tonic to the digestion. **Ginger** acts as a stimulant; its warming action is good for the atonic state.

DIETARY AND OTHER ADVICE

The patient is advised to eat a regular whole-food diet; little and often at first (avoiding eating late, drinking coffee and especially fry-ups and cheese). He should take regular

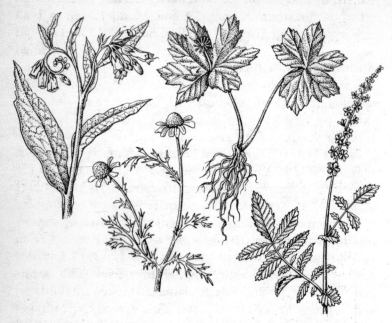

Comfrey, Golden Seal

exercise, and practise deep-breathing exercises. If possible, he should take a holiday.

Chinese-style herbalist

ANALYSIS: (see Appendix B)
The chronic nature of the complaint, with its dull pain (which feels better on pressure), combined with tiredness, pale tongue and weak pulse, points to this being a deficient condition. The fact that pain is relieved by warm drinks, and that the tongue has a white coat, suggests a cold condition. Nausea and belching (rebellious stomach Qi) indicate stomach derangement. Loss of appetite, tiredness,

pallor and occasional diarrhoea indicate spleen Qi deficiency.*

SUMMARY
The patient is deficient and cold in spleen and stomach.

PREDISPOSING CAUSES
As for western herbalist.

STRATEGY
Tonify spleen and stomach Qi; warm the cold.

PRESCRIPTION
The prescription used in this case is called the *Xiang Sha:* Six Gentlemen Soup, a recipe which dates back to the Song dynasty, around AD 1200.

Costus root (*Saussurea lappa*) 3 gm
Grains of paradise (*Amomum villosum*) 3 gm
Ginseng (*Panax ginseng*) 6 gm
White atractylodes (*Atractylodes macrocephala*) 6 gm
Poria (*Poria cocos*) 6 gm
Citrus peel (*Citrus reticulata*) 3 gm
Pinellia (*Pinellia ternata*) 6 gm
Honey-baked liquorice (*Glycyrrhiza uralensis*) 3 gm

Boil for half an hour in 1½ litres of water and strain. Drink one cupful, warm, after meals, three times a day.

ANALYSIS OF PRESCRIPTION
Costus root moves the Qi and alleviates pain. Strengthens the spleen. Warming. **Grains of paradise** warm the stomach and spleen, stopping diarrhoea. Reduces nausea. **Ginseng** tonifies the spleen Qi. It is used for tiredness,

* In Chinese medicine, the spleen has different functions to those ascribed to it by western medicine. Traditional Chinese 'physiology' pairs the spleen (yin organ) with the stomach (yang organ) to govern, among other things, the digestive function. While stomach energy, or Qi, goes downwards in health – thus rebellious stomach Qi causes belching, nausea and vomiting – healthy spleen Qi goes upwards. Derangement of this can lead to diarrhoea (the spleen Qi fails to hold the stools), and heaviness and fatigue.

diarrhoea, lack of appetite and vomiting if associated with deficient spleen Qi (as here). Warming. **White atractylodes** tonifies spleen Qi. Warming. **Poria** reinforces Qi of spleen and stomach. **Citrus peel** tonifies and regulates spleen Qi; invigorates the appetite; counters nausea and belching. Warming. Blends other ingredients. **Pinellia** is good for nausea and phlegm. Warming. **Liquorice** acts as in western prescriptions. Liquorice also blends and harmonizes all the other ingredients in the prescription. Honey-baked liquorice used by the Chinese herbalist, is thought better for helping digestive problems.

If the patient still complains of tiredness, **Astragalus** (*Astragalus membranaceus*) may be added to this remedy. Astragalus tonifies the spleen and benefits the Qi and, like ginseng, is very useful for debilitated states.

DIETARY AND OTHER ADVICE
The patient is advised not to eat cold or fried food (i.e. advice as given by the western herbalist).

Case 2

Margaret X; fifty-eight years old. She has suffered pain and stiffness in her knees and ankles for the last four years, which is gradually getting worse, especially during damp and cold weather. The symptoms improved considerably during a previous summer holiday in Spain, and are temporarily relieved by hot baths. They are, however, made worse by climbing stairs and long periods of standing (now that her three children have grown up she has resumed her career as a librarian). She likes gardening, which is her only exercise, but finds this increasingly difficult. In all other respects she is healthy and has suffered no serious illness. She enjoys life. She is somewhat overweight and tends not to take a lot of trouble over her diet, beyond intermittent bouts of slimming. She usually has just a cup of coffee for breakfast, sandwiches at lunchtime, and a full meal (meat and vegetables) for supper. Confesses a weakness for biscuits, cake and chocolate. Does not drink or smoke.

X-rays of her knees showed no discernible joint changes. Her GP prescribed Brufen, which helped alleviate the pain and stiffness, but she does not want to continue taking the drug on a long-term basis.

Examination

There is loss of mobility, and pain on flexing knees. Slight crepitus (grating of the joint) audible. Slight swelling of the left knee (the more painful of the two), and definite puffiness of the skin of the lower limbs and around the ankles. The skin feels a little moist. Blood pressure, and all other examinations, revealed no other abnormalities. The tongue has a pale body with a slightly thick white coat. The pulse is soft and rather weak.

Western herbalist

ANALYSIS
Osteoarthritis, as a result of poor tissue drainage and circulation, shown by puffy, oedematous skin. The knees and ankles, being weight-bearing joints, are under strain due to the patient being overweight.

PREDISPOSING CAUSES
Exposure to cold, damp weather conditions and too much standing.

STRATEGY
Drain the tissues of their toxic-waste build-up; stimulate the circulation and reduce inflammation.

PRESCRIPTION

Begin by taking, for two weeks, a herbal infusion, while also observing dietary and other recommendations (see below).

Equal parts of:
    Horsetail (*Equisetum arvense*)
    Cornsilk (*Zea mays*)   } as an infusion
    Nettles (*Urtica dioica*)

Dosage: one wineglassful three times a day.

After two weeks reduce this dosage to twice daily, and take the following tincture:

Tinctures of:

Celery seed (*Apium graveolens*)	10 ml
Burdock (*Arctium lappa*)	15 ml
Dandelion root (*Taraxacum officinale*)	10 ml
Meadowsweet (*Filipendula ulmaria*)	15 ml
Devil's claw (*Harpagophytum procumbens*)	20 ml
Sarsaparilla (*Smilax spp*)	20 ml
Prickly ash (*Xanthoxylum americanum*)	10 ml
	———
	100 ml

After meals, three times a day, take a teaspoon of tincture, diluted in warm water.

In addition, during the day the patient can use a cabbage poultice on her knees, which stimulates circulation to the painful area. The cabbage leaf should be bruised before application and held in place with a knee-support bandage. At night the patient is asked to use a comfrey poultice consisting of:

                Comfrey leaves 6 parts
                Powdered slippery elm 9 parts
                Lobelia 3 parts
                Cayenne 1 part

Add 90 gm of the mixture to hot water to make a paste. Spread the paste on a cloth and apply to affected area.

The patient is also advised to make use of footbaths. The feet are soaked in this bath for ten minutes before going to bed.

Footbath:
  30 gm fresh ginger root
  2 cinnamon sticks

Simmer in 600 ml of water for fifteen minutes. Strain. Add the decoction to 1500 ml of hot water, and dissolve into this 270 gm of Epsom salts (which are cheaper when bought as magnesium sulphate crystals). The water for this bath can be re-heated and re-used for about six days provided it is stored somewhere cool.

EXPLANATION OF THE PRESCRIPTION

The preliminary infusion is used to get rid of excess fluid and waste materials before using deeper detoxifying remedies like devil's claw and sarsaparilla to release more wastes from the tissues. This infusion will activate and strengthen the kidneys to do their depurative work and avoid a crisis as the deeper remedies begin to act. Diuretic herbal remedies work best as infusions.

Cornsilk and **horsetail** are both diuretics, strengthening the kidneys. **Nettles** help to rid the body of harmful excess acids. **Celery seed** stimulates the elimination of uric acid and has a diuretic effect. **Burdock** is a diuretic which has a deep-cleansing effect on the tissues. **Dandelion root** acts as a bitter tonic to the digestion, as well as being a mild diuretic and liver cleanser. It also helps to purify the blood and tissues. **Meadowsweet** contains salicylic glycosides, giving it an anti-inflammatory action. It is also diuretic. **Devil's claw** is a remedy indigenous to South and East Africa, with a deserved reputation for reducing inflammation and detoxifying the body. Scientific tests show that this herb compares favourably with the effects of a commonly used anti-inflammatory drug, phenylbutazone. **Sarsaparilla** is another deep detoxifying remedy. It is gently stimulating to the circulation. **Prickly ash** is a circulatory stimulant, increasing blood flow to the tissues. This remedy also has proven anti-inflammatory action.

DIETARY AND OTHER ADVICE

Dietary change is important. The diet should consist of whole grains and alkalinizing fresh vegetables, including warming and stimulating foods like cabbage, turnip, watercress and radish, as well as spices like garlic, ginger and horseradish. All sour and acid fruits, especially rhubarb, citrus fruits and pickles, are to be avoided. For this reason, the patient should also reduce the intake of tomatoes. Red meats are to be avoided; chicken (free-range) and fresh fish can be eaten instead. The patient is advised to eat breakfast and avoid cakes, biscuits and chocolates. She is asked not to drink coffee, substituting it with herbal teas and mineral water.

Exercise is recommended, in moderation, especially swimming and walking.

Chinese herbalist

ANALYSIS

This is a case of cold, damp *bi* syndrome. *Bi*, in Chinese, means blockage, and here the channels or meridians which carry the Qi and blood to the lower limbs are blocked by an invasion of damp and cold. Dampness is a yin evil, and sinks, often causing problems in the lower part of the body. Coldness causes contraction (stiffness) and pain. Puffiness and swelling and moist skin are also signs of dampness.

The strength of the lower back and legs is consequent on the patient's healthy kidneys, whose energy may be damaged by too much lifting or standing. However, except for the arthritis, the patient is well; this is primarily a disease of the channels rather than of the internal organs.

A soft pulse is characteristic of damp conditions, as is a thick tongue coat. The white colour of the coat confirms the cold condition. The weakness of the pulse and the pale tongue show the underlying condition is one of deficiency.

PREDISPOSING CAUSES
As for western herbalist.

STRATEGY
Expel cold and dampness; tonify and move the Qi and blood.

PRESCRIPTION
The Chinese herbalist uses an ancient prescription called the Pubescent Angelica and Loranthus Decoction (*Du Huo Ji Sheng Tang*):

> Pubescent angelica (*Angelica pubescens*) 6 gm
> Large-leaf gentian (*Gentiana macrophylla*) 3 gm
> Ledebouriella (*Ledebouriella seseloides*) 3gm
> Wild ginger (*Asarum sieboldii*) 2 gm
> Mulberry mistletoe (*Loranthus parasiticus*) 6 gm
> Eucommia (*Eucommia ulmoides*) 3 gm
> Achyranthes (*Achyranthes bidentata*) 3 gm
> Cinnamon twigs (*Cinnamomum cassia*) 2 gm
> Chinese angelica (*Angelica sinensis*) 3 gm
> Chinese lovage (*Ligusticum wallichii*) 3 gm
> Rehmannia root (*Rehmannia glutinosa*) 6 gm
> White peony (*Paeonia lactiflora*) 3 gm
> Codonopsis (*Codonopsis pilosula*) 3 gm
> Poria (*Poria cocos*) 9 gm
> Liquorice (*Glycyrrhiza uralensis*) 3 gm

Boil for twenty minutes in 2 litres of water. Strain and drink warm; one cup three times a day before meals.

ANALYSIS OF PRESCRIPTION

Because it has fifteen herbs, this prescription may at first seem rather unwieldy, but further study shows it to be composed rather like a well-scored piece of music, with each instrument playing an important role.

Three of its herbs are famous for driving out dampness: **pubescent angelica** (used especially for the lower part of the body), **large-leaf gentian** and **ledebouriella**. **Wild ginger** and **cinnamon twigs** warm the meridians and expel cold. Three herbs tonify the kidneys: **achyranthes** (especially good for pain in the lower back and knees); **mulberry mistletoe** (which also gets rid of dampness and tonifies the blood); and **eucommia** (which helps to move stagnant Qi and blood). Another three all tonify the Qi: **codonopsis**; **poria** (which has a diuretic action); and **liquorice** (which also harmonizes the whole prescription). The final four herbs – **rehmannia** (prepared), **Chinese angelica**, **Chinese lovage** and **white peony** – compose the famous Four Ingredients Decoction (*Si Wu Tang*), renowned for tonifying the blood and regulating its circulation.

The combination of cinnamon and peony is famous for driving out external evils which have penetrated into the channels, harmonizing the *Ying* (internal) and *Wei* (external) *Qi*.

DIETARY AND OTHER ADVICE

As for the western herbalist – avoid sour foods; eat regularly. Avoid kneeling on damp ground or otherwise getting wet while gardening.

Case 3

Mary X; twenty-seven years old. Asthma since she was nineteen, when she worked as a seed consultant, visiting farms. As a child she had hayfever. Her asthma is worse in the summer months, aggravated by cigarette-smoke, horses, cats and dust. Acute attacks have been controlled by using Becotide and Ventolin inhalers, but she still wheezes when she is excited or anxious (she admits to being 'a worrier') and when she takes exercise. As a child, her mother also had asthma but 'grew out of it'. Her two year old daughter has eczema and 'is a bit wheezy'. She is happily married and remembers her childhood with affection.

Examination

Wheezing clearly audible. The patient is thin and anxious. She holds herself tensely, which is consistent with her comments about worrying. Tongue, red with a yellow, slightly sticky coat. Pulse, rapid and slightly slippery. Phlegm, sticky, yellow.

Western herbalist

ANALYSIS
Asthma of allergic origin? Probably, since it was triggered by contact with grasses and cereals in the course of her work (she already was allergic, as shown by her regular bouts of hay fever). It looks as if this is an inherited problem.

STRATEGY
Treat the asthma by relaxing the airways, and treat the whole person by relaxing and strengthening the nervous system. Use elimination diets to try to identify any particular allergen or food sensitivity.

PRESCRIPTION

Pillbearing spurge (*Euphorbia pilulifera*)	15	ml
Grindelia (*Grindelia camporum*)	15	ml
Ephedra (Ma huang, *Ephedra sinica*)	7.5	ml
Lobelia (*Lobelia inflata*)	5	ml
Ginger (*Zingiber officinale*)	5	ml
Liquorice (*Glycyrrhiza glabra*)	7.5	ml
Skunk cabbage (*Symplocarpus foetidus*)	15	ml
Coltsfoot (*Tussilago farfara*)	15	ml
Cowslip (*Primula veris*)	15	ml
	100	ml

Take a teaspoon of the tincture, diluted in warm water, three to four times a day. The use of a vapourizer, to diffuse oils of pine or lavender into the air while sleeping, is also recommended.

EXPLANATION OF THE PRESCRIPTION

Pillbearing spurge, grindelia, ephedra and **lobelia** are all bronchial relaxants and expectorants. **Ginger** acts as a stimulating, warming remedy, combining well with lobelia and increasing the duration of its effect. So although the patient presents an over-stimulated picture, this remedy is still applicable. **Liquorice** is an expectorant and demulcent. It has a strengthening effect on the adrenal glands, which are under stress in asthmatic patients. **Skunk cabbage** relaxes the airways and an overstressed nervous system. **Coltsfoot** is a good general expectorant. **Cowslip** has a dual action as an expectorant, while gently relaxing the nervous system too.

DIETARY AND OTHER ADVICE

This patient is asked to follow a wheat, dairy and egg-free diet* for three weeks, recording all she eats and drinks, and

---

* These foods are common allergens. Here wheat is particularly suspect because of the previous history of hay fever.

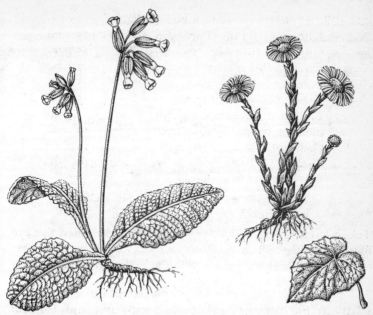

Cowslip, coltsfoot

also keeping a record of her symptoms and how often she needs her inhalers. Her general diet turns out to be good, requiring little change. She is asked, however, to avoid dried fruits and alcohol, which may contain sulphur dioxide, since this is known to trigger asthma attacks. After three weeks she will return to her diet the foods she is avoiding, one by one, to see if there is any change.

It is recommended that she practises abdominal breathing exercises each day and considers taking up singing, which is beneficial for asthmatics. She is also asked to take gentle exercise.

Chinese herbalist

ANALYSIS

The wheezing and shortness of breath indicate a lung problem. The rapid pulse, red tongue-body and yellow tongue-coat indicate heat. The slippery pulse and sticky tongue-coating indicate phlegm. The diagnosis is retention of phlegm-heat in the lung.

STRATEGY
Clear heat and resolve phlegm. Tonify the lungs.

PRESCRIPTION
Use the Stabilize Asthma Soup (*Ding Chuan Tang*)

> Ginkgo seed (*Ginkgo biloba*) 2 pieces
> Ma huang (*Ephedra sinica*) 3 gm
> Perilla seed (*Perilla frutescens*) 8 gm
> Coltsfoot (*Tussilago farfara*) 8 gm
> Apricot seed (*Prunus armeniaca*) 8 gm
> Mulberry bark (*Morus alba*) 8 gm
> Skullcap root (*Scutellaria baicalensis*) 4 gm
> Pinellia (*Pinellia ternata*) 8 gm
> Liquorice (*Glycyrrhiza uralensis*) 3 gm

To this traditional prescription we add one herb:

> Peucedanum (*Peucedanum praeruptorum*) 4 gm

Boil for twenty minutes in 2 litres of water. Strain and drink warm, one cup three times a day, before meals.

ANALYSIS OF PRESCRIPTION
This prescription shows a neat balance between warming and cooling herbs. Although the overall requirement is to 'clear heat', the presence of warming herbs, like ma huang, perilla, coltsfoot, apricot and pinellia, which help the breathing, is balanced by the cooling effect of the mulberry bark, scullcap root, and the addition of peucedanum. The scullcap root is particularly important for reducing heat in the lungs. Pinellia is famous for removing phlegm. Liquorice is harmonizing, and the remaining herbs stop coughing and relieve asthma.

DIETARY AND OTHER ADVICE

The patient is asked to eat cooling foods, and avoid hot, spicy, greasy food, and alcohol.

CHAPTER FOUR

CONSULTATION

So far we have looked at herbal treatment from the practitioner's point of view, but what is it like to be a herbal patient?

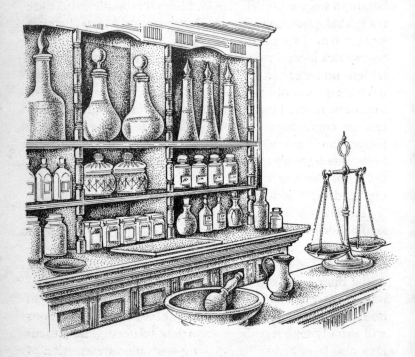

There are no broomsticks, black cats or bubbling cauldrons in the herbalist's consulting room or dispensary. A herbal surgery is, in many respects, no different from a GP's surgery, usually having a desk or table at which the practitioner sits, and a chair for the patient. There are also other items in the room, which one would expect to see in a doctor's surgery: an examination couch, stethoscope, sphygmomanometer (to measure blood pressure), ophthalmoscope and auriscope (to examine the eyes and ears), patellar hammer (to test reflexes) and so on. These are as much the professional herbalist's tools of trade as they are the doctor's.

There will, however, probably be some differences between the herbal surgery and that of the orthodox doctor. Although, due to public demand, some chemists have begun to stock a limited range of herbal remedies, there are no herbal pharmacies in the high street. Most chemists who, two or three generations ago, could have been counted on to stock a good range of herbal tinctures, ointments and tablets, no longer do so. For this reason, nearly all herbalists have their own pharmacy. The sight of rows of bottles of tinctures, neatly labelled in Latin (common English names can be confusing), or bottles of dried herbs, greet the patient coming into the clinic. Outside the surgery, many herbalists have a herb garden in which they grow some of the herbs they use in their practice. Here marigolds, hyssop, sage and vervain also welcome the patients as they arrive.

Herbalists who are members of reputable professional associations are not permitted to advertise, so it is likely that the first appointment is made as a result of a recommendation by a friend, relation or colleague. When the initial phone call is made, the patient will be given an appointment time and, as a rule, will be asked to allow an hour for this first consultation. Subsequent consultations will usually take less time, according to need. The patient may also be asked to bring along a detailed description of what he or she eats (this can be done by keeping a diet-diary for four or five days), plus any relevant medical records, X-rays, results of blood and urine tests, and so on.

In practice, herbal treatment is hardly ever available on the N H S. The first consultation usually costs from ten to twenty pounds, while subsequent appointments may vary from five to fifteen pounds, depending on how long they take. Medicines usually cost around an additional two pounds a week. These figures are obviously only a rough

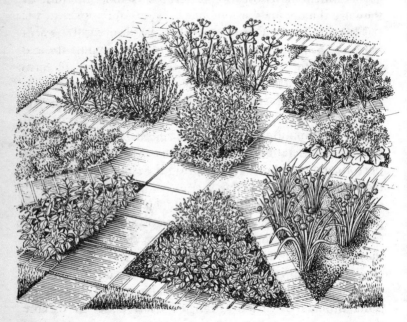

The herb garden

guide. Special rates are usually available for OAP's and the unwaged. Some private health-insurance schemes may reimburse the cost of herbal treatment, if it has the blessing of a hospital consultant.

Since herbal treatment is 'low tech', and far cheaper than its orthodox counterpart, it is looking increasingly attractive to health-insurance companies; it seems only a matter of time before herbal treatments get medical-insurance backing. It is also hoped that one day herbal treatment can become part of State-funded medicine, as it is in several

Third World countries like China and India. It would save the NHS millions of pounds presently spent on drugs.

The reason why the initial consultation takes at least an hour is because, during this time, the herbalist needs to gather an enormous amount of information about the patient. The consultation starts from the moment the patient and practitioner meet – a great deal can be learnt from the tone of someone's voice, from their posture and gait, eyes and face (its colour and expression). A firm handshake, for instance, immediately suggests that here is plenty of vital force, while, on a cool day, a perceptibly wet or shaky hand could indicate nervousness, or even poor urinary elimination. Throughout the consultation, clues are gradually pieced together to construct a picture of the whole person, and the herbal prescription is designed accordingly like a close-fitting garment.

During this initial meeting the herbalist will ask the patient many questions that a GP might also ask. For example, what is the problem that brings you here? How long has it troubled you? How and when did it start? How frequently does it occur? Are there associated problems? If there is pain, what is its character and location? And so on. This process of enquiry can be quite a strain on the memory, so it is a good idea if, before coming to see the herbalist, the patient makes notes about what he or she wants to discuss. This way nothing gets forgotten. Remembering one's medical and family history is also important; these details help the herbalist to establish the context of the present problems, and the overall state of health. Although a previous illness may no longer seem relevant, it can sometimes point to a fundamental weakness that must be redressed before full health can be restored. During herbal treatment of a chronic problem, it can happen that symptoms of previous illnesses, which were not properly treated at the time, may recur for a while and then be resolved. This is a healthy process; the body and mind have an unconscious memory of everything experienced, and this can reflect on our present lives in ways of which we are not consciously aware. For this reason the herbalist will want to know all about previous medication, as well as any drugs currently being taken.

The herbalist will be interested in the patient as a person, not just in the particular problem that he or she has come about. Relevant questions about the emotional, mental and spiritual well-being of a patient may have to wait for a second or third meeting, when a rapport between patient and practitioner has been struck up. All consultations are, of course, in strict confidence, and a good herbalist will never force the pace in assessing any rather more private aspects. It is important, for the success of the treatment, that the herbalist does have time for the patient, and listens sympathetically as well as giving advice. Even an arthritic knee can feel better when some long-held worry or fear has been brought out into the open. In this way, the treatment begins before the first dose of herbal medicine is taken.

The food diary comes in useful here too, because the herbal practitioner will want to know all about what the patient usually eats. A balanced, whole-food diet (with its full quota of vitamins, trace-elements and minerals) is vital for maintaining good health. Some ailments can be remedied just by healthy eating, or by special diets. In treating more serious health problems, foods are still an important aid to herbal treatment. There is no clear demarcation between medicinal herbs and fruits and vegetables, many of which – for example, cherries, walnuts, celery, cabbage, asparagus, corn, lettuce, carrots and onions – have clear medicinal properties.

Knowledge of the therapeutic use of food is thousands of years old. For instance, the Yellow Emperor's *Classic of Internal Medicine* recommended 'bitter food to drain the spleen, and sweet food to supplement and strengthen it', while it advised 'sour food to supplement and strengthen the lungs but pungent food to drain them and make them expel'. The American Indians also knew a thing or two about diet. During the bitter winter of 1535–6, an expedition of three ships, led by Jacques Cartier, became ice-bound in the St Lawrence river. The crew, who lived on the preserved foods and hard tack from the holds of their ships, became extremely ill, and soon nearly a quarter of them had died of scurvy. Cartier however was fortunate to get help from a local Indian chief, who gave the survivors a tea of the green needles of the black spruce, rich in Vitamin C. More than two hundred years later, British naval surgeon James Lind, who read about Cartier's experience, did some experiments which proved the dietary basis of scurvy.

Herbal practitioners follow Hippocrates' advice: 'Let foods be your medicine.' Nearly two thousand years later Dr Lyle, the physiomedical herbalist, wrote:

In the treatment of disease, make your patient's food subservient to your medication. Then both food and medicine will become instrumental under the vital force in the restorative act. Some foods are stimulating in their nature, as beef, beets, cranberries, parsley, sour apples, rhubarb. Some foods are astringent as boiled milk, fine flour, crab apples, arrowroot. Some foods are relaxing to the system as turnips, sweet apples, asparagus.[1]

The health-giving or detrimental properties of foods are common knowledge in China. For instance, Chinese women know to avoid cold foods and drinks during menstruation because these may cause painful periods. I well remember at the breakfast-banquet which was my farewell party at the Chinese hospital where I had been studying, the hospital director (an administrator, not a doctor) went through every item of food and drink on the table, describing the medicinal value of each one. As we have seen, both Chinese and Ayurvedic medicine define the medicinal action of herbs by their temperature and taste, and these same energetic criteria are also used to evaluate food. Chinese herb doctors, perceiving that someone has a cold disease, may prescribe warming foods like carp, beef, lamb, venison, pigeon, wheat, broad beans, ginger and onions. A patient suffering from a hot condition, on the other hand, would be advised to avoid such food and instead eat cooling foods such as crab, turtle, rabbit, pears, water melon, lettuce, bamboo shoots, tomatoes and cucumber (cf Culpeper's famous remark about cucumber: 'If it were but one degree colder, it would be a poison').

The herbal practitioner may suggest changes to the patient's diet, sometimes also eliminating certain foods for a time because of suspected allergies. Allergies seem to be on the increase. This is probably due to the many artificial chemical additives in commercial foods, as well as agricultural sprays. Orthodox drugs can also undermine the strength of the body's immune system; even the loss of so many healthy men in two world wars has contributed towards weakening the human gene-pool.

After a full case-history has been taken, the herbalist will need to examine the patient. This may mean taking the pulse and blood pressure, looking at the tongue, and checking over each of the body's systems in turn, using gentle palpation and percussion and diagnostic tools like a stethoscope. During the examination, apart from trying to identify specific pathological problems, the herbalist will also be assessing the general tone (or lack of it) of the skin, muscles, digestion, circulatory and nervous systems. This overall view is invaluable. An overcontracted small intestine can generally be palpated by the examining hand, while the drum-like (tympanic) tone of the bowel area may indicate an over-relaxed colon, each state calling for different herbal remedies. Similarly, while brisk tendon reflexes can indicate disease of the nervous system, in the absence of other signs and symptoms such a finding may be a valuable clue to a merely overstressed nervous system. Here the herbalist might prescribe nervine relaxants (like passion flower and lady's slipper) together with a nervous restorative (like wild oats), to restore the balance. As well as examining the patient, the herbalist may wish to do simple clinical tests such as urine analysis.

Many people visiting herbalists for the first time are on medication from the doctor. The herbalist will certainly not act irresponsibly by advising the dropping of vital drugs until it is clear that the patient can do without them. Where possible the patient is asked to talk over any change in medication with his or her own doctor. Many patients come to see a herbalist because they cannot cope with the side-effects of the drugs they are taking. Some are hopelessly addicted to tranquillizers and sedatives, which are often harder to give up than heroin. According to Professor Malcolm Lader of the Institute of Psychiatry, tranquillizers are ineffective after four months and sleeping pills become useless after a fortnight. He estimates that around a quarter of a million people are dependent on benzodiazepines (the drugs concerned). Herbal medicines can be helpful to wean someone off these kinds of pills.

Herbal treatment usually requires that the patient actively participates in the work of getting better, rather than just taking a drug and surrendering responsibility for this process. Aside from dietary work, it may be important, for the success of the treatment, that the patient gets more exercise, or practises relaxation or deep breathing exercises to counter stress and bring peace of mind. The herbal practitioner may also encourage the use of positive visualization techniques, which help to mobilize the healing power of the body and overcome fears and inadequacies. In this way the patient and practitioner work together – partners with a common goal.

A difference between herbal and orthodox medical

treatment is the time factor. Today people have come to expect rapid (if not instant) results from taking medicines. Drugs are concentrated, powerful chemicals which act rapidly on the body, but herbs are much more gentle. If one uses herbs in the holistic way described earlier, it may (though not always) take several months for a chronic health problem to ease. In acute disease, healing may often be much more rapid. The healing that takes place is real, not symptomatic, and its side-effect is that there is an increased feeling of well-being. (Herbs, of course, can also be used to maintain good health, by drinking herb teas and including culinary herbs in cooking.) So the call on the patient is to be just this – *patient*. In general, the longer a person has been ill, the longer the cure. A very rough guide would be to allow a month of treatment for each year the problem has existed.

The number of consultations this involves will vary. Usually there will be a second meeting fairly soon after the initial one, say in about a fortnight's time. This would mainly be used to check that the medicine has been well tolerated, and to discuss how dietary changes or exercise, etc., are going. Subsequent meetings may occur at monthly intervals, depending on the case. At each consultation the herbalist has an opportunity to adjust the herbal medicine to suit the changing needs of the patient.

Some people have constitutional weaknesses which may always predispose them to a particular kind of problem, and here herbal treatment may be required from time to time for years rather than months.

Healing crises can be a feature of herbal treatment. We have already discussed how former health problems may recur for a time during a course of treatment. This is one kind of healing crisis. Another is when the body's power becomes strong enough to deal with a chronic problem in a more active way, and there can be an apparent flare-up of symptoms for a few days. For example, there may be an increase for a short while in the pain of an arthritic joint. The herbalist will use all his or her skill to prevent this from being too drastic, but such exacerbations are a good sign, and we always warn our patients to look out for them and not to worry if they happen. Characteristically, such healing crises last only a short while and after they have resolved themselves the patient feels much improved.

Sometimes it happens that a patient has need of special medical investigations or treatment that is beyond the scope of herbal medicine. In such a case the herbalist will ask the patient to visit his or her doctor or specialist. This occurred recently when I discovered that a patient, who had come to see me complaining of headaches, had dangerously high blood pressure. I asked him to immediately go to see his doctor and within twenty-four hours he was being operated on for a tumour on the adrenal glands, which was responsible for the rise in blood pressure and his headaches. In this case herbal treatment could have done nothing for the patient except dangerously delay the required operation.

Patients sometimes conceal from their doctor the fact that they are visiting a herbalist for fear of what the doctor might say. This is a shame because doctors and herbalists ought to work together. The two kinds of medicine are complementary. It is certainly true that a decade or so ago the majority of doctors were prejudiced against alternative or complementary medicine, but now many doctors do acknowledge its possible benefit.*

---

* A survey (the results of which were published in the *British Medical Journal*, 30 July 1983), conducted amongst one hundred G P-trainees, showed that eighteen already used at least one alternative therapy; no fewer than seventy would like to have training in one or more; while twenty-two either had been treated or had treated themselves with an alternative therapy.

People often ask what diseases herbalists treat. Herbalists do not treat diseases – they treat people. Some diseases may be 'incurable', but herbal medicine can still help to raise the level of general health in someone suffering from, say Parkinson's disease or multiple sclerosis – even when a cure cannot be expected. To give some kind of indication of the range of herbal treatment, however, here is a list of some of the problems which herbalists may treat.

Colds, coughs, flu, tonsillitis and many other infectious diseases, children's ailments.

Bronchitis, asthma, sinusitis and catarrh, hayfever.

Indigestion, hiatus hernia, gastritis, gastric and duodenal ulcers, gallstones, irritable bowel disease, diverticulitis, haemorrhoids, constipation, diarrhoea.

Poor circulation, chilblains, varicose veins and ulcers, palpitations, angina, high and low blood pressure.

Headaches and migraines, stress, anxiety and depression, insomnia, lassitude.

Eczema, psoriasis, cold sores, shingles, fungal infections, boils.

Pre-menstrual tension, painful periods, lack of periods, endometriosis, menopausal problems, infertility, breast-feeding problems, preparation for pregnancy and child-birth, baby's colic, post-natal depression, prostate problems.

Cystitis, kidney infections, kidney stones.

Arthritis and gout, muscular tension.

Allergies and drug withdrawal.

Lists of illnesses should not obscure, for both herbalist and patient, the central issues of disease. There is an old Latin saying: '*Medicus curat, natura sanat*' – the doctor treats but nature heals. Ultimately healing comes not from medicines, whether drugs or herbs, but from the innate wisdom and strength of our true nature. Moreover we can, and should, learn from disease. The lessons and achievements of life come through struggle, and disease is part of this process. At its simplest level, illness can tell us that we are eating unwisely, or not taking enough exercise. It can also help us to change more fundamentally. Negative emotional or mental attitudes will also predispose us towards particular illnesses. For example, someone who worries too much may suffer from headaches. In such cases, for real healing to take place, a deep change must occur. Afterwards the person will be wiser and stronger. 'Medicine' which merely knocks out or suppresses symptoms ultimately does us no favours at all. The problems we do not confront today can contribute to trouble later on because our innate wisdom will try to make us face up to and work on our weaknesses in some other way.

We need to learn how to embrace our sickness, not to fear it. Perhaps this fear comes ultimately from a fear of death, but death itself can be a creative, developing process. Sometimes the best treatment helps people to die positively, without fear, even with joy.

CHAPTER FIVE

HERB AID

There is surely no better way to gain confidence in herbal medicine than to use it oneself. This section suggests just a few simple yet effective herbal treatments for minor emergencies. Here herbs can be a valuable substitute for expensive, over-the-counter medicines. Many of the herbs recommended can provide double service, their colour and aroma being a welcome addition to a garden of any size. Culinary herbs like mint, thyme, rosemary and sage, which can be grown in a garden and used as medicines, also add an irreplaceable dimension to one's cooking.

Before the introduction of the NHS, many people relied on herbs for medicines because they could not afford the services of a doctor, or the cost of drugs. Country people had a good working knowledge of the remedies which could be made up of the herbs that grew around them. Whenever the legislators tried to quash the practice of herbal medicine, they quickly discovered its enormous popularity. We saw in Chapter 1 how unsuccessful Henry VIII was when he tried to prevent ordinary people from getting herbal treatment. Today herbal medicine remains the people's medicine. In 1941 there was a huge public outcry when the wartime government (which surely should have had better things to do with its time!) with indecent haste rushed into law the Pharmacy and Medicines Act, which in effect made the practice of herbal medicine by trained herbal practitioners illegal.*

* When it came to framing the 1968 Medicines Act (passed in the wake of the thalidomide disaster) the government, it seems, had learnt the lesson of the furore caused by the 1941 Act, and so determined to reverse it by making special provision in the new Act to allow for the legitimate practice of herbal medicine.

A recent survey shows that of all forms of alternative medicine, herbal medicine appears to be the most popular. So despite the advances of modern medicine, people have not given up their allegiance to it.*

There is only one danger with herbal self-medication: one may get out of one's depth, and perhaps delay having some serious ailment treated by a professional. If you are at all unsure about what the problem is, or how to treat it, or if it lasts any more than a day or two without improvement, it is vital that you immediately seek the advice of a herbal practitioner or doctor (or perhaps where appropriate some other trained alternative therapist).

General information in the preparation of herbal medicine is given in Chapter 7.

Common cold

The common cold is just that – *common*. Can there be anyone who does not have first-hand experience of its all too familiar symptoms? Colds are caused by viruses, which hide away inside the body's cells and so cannot be destroyed by antibiotic drugs – such drugs only kill the bacteria that live outside the protection of the cell walls. Herbal treatment, on the other hand, aims to strengthen the body's own natural defences so that a cold can be nipped in the bud.

At the onset of the first chills heralding a cold, take this decoction, which is made from kitchen spices:

* The 1984 survey carried out by the independent research body RSGB revealed that twelve per cent of a sample of two thousand people had tried herbal medicine (more than any other alternative therapy). Seventy-three per cent reported that they were satisfied with the treatment. A more recent *Which?* report (October 1986) declared that of the people in their survey who had visited a herbalist, nearly a quarter claimed to have been cured, and nearly half said they had improved. Nearly eight out of ten said they would use a herbalist again.

> Fresh ginger root 30 gm (sliced)
> Cinnamon sticks 1–2 (broken up)
> Coriander seeds 2.5 gm
> Cloves 4
> Water 600 ml

Bring to the boil, cover the pan and simmer for twenty minutes. In the last five minutes add a slice of lemon. Strain and sweeten with organic honey to taste. Drink a cupful, hot, every two to three hours.

Alternatively, make a tea comprising in equal parts:

> Hyssop
> Elderflowers   } to make 30 gm
> Mint (any type)

Pour 500 ml of boiling water on to this mixture; cover (to avoid loss of volatile oils) and let it stand for ten to fifteen minutes. Strain and drink a cupful, hot, every hour or so.

Commercial preparations

Composition Essence (physiomedical formula). Use 1–2 teaspoons to a cup of hot water. Drink frequently. Good for colds with chills.

Jade Screen Powder. A Chinese formula available from Chinese pharmacies. This formula strengthens the body's defensive energy (*Wei Qi*). Good for those who suffer from constantly recurring colds.

Foods and supplements

For Vitamin C, which boosts the body's immune system, eat plenty of oranges, and drink rose-hip tea, and hot lemon and honey. Take 1–3 gm a day of natural Vitamin C. Select warming foods such as garlic, green onions (also known as scallions or spring onions) or the common onion. All are best eaten raw. Add cayenne pepper to food. Also helpful

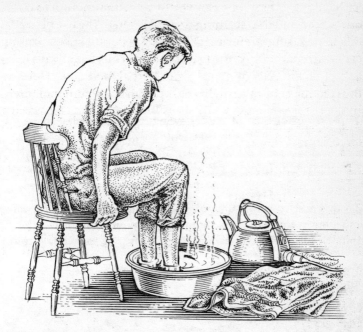

Mustard footbaths are an effective way to treat the common cold

to combat a cold are watercress, cabbage, black pepper and mustard. A mustard footbath is worth trying. Make this by putting a dessertspoon of mustard powder in 1 litre of hot water, and bathing the feet in it for around eight minutes, before going to bed. Avoid mucus-forming foods like dairy products and eggs.

Catarrh

Colds are often accompanied by catarrh. This may be alleviated by inhaling volatile oils in steam. Such inhalations are made by pouring boiling water over herbs or oils, and making a 'tent' of a cloth or towel, large enough to cover one's head and the steaming bowl. Although the use of herbal oils is now sometimes regarded as a separate specialization called aromatherapy, the use of essential oils has always been an important part of mainstream herbal medicine. Here, in the treatment of catarrh, herbal oils can come into their own.

Three drops of each of the following oils in a bowl:

> Eucalyptus
> Peppermint
> Pine
> Wintergreen

To this add 10 ml of tincture of benzoin. Boil 500 ml of water and allow it to stand for a minute before pouring it into the bowl. Inhale. This mixture, using just one drop of each oil, 5 ml of

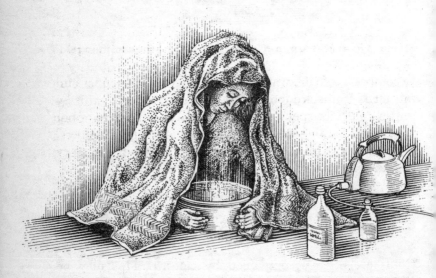

Steam inhalations are good for coughs, colds and sinus problems

tincture of benzoin and less water, can be put into a simple vapourizer (available from chemists), which can be burnt at night, filling the bedroom with its healing, antiseptic vapours.

Commercial preparation

Olbas oil.

Foods

A fruit-fast is excellent for one to three days. As in the case of a cold, avoid mucus-forming foods like dairy products. Drink mint or thyme tea. Eat garlic, onions, and add oregano, ginger and cayenne pepper to cooking. The Chinese also caution against eating mushrooms during a cold.

Sore throat

Gargle:

> Sage leaves (dried or fresh) 1 handful
> Boiling water 500 ml

Pour the boiling water on the herb and cover. Let it stand until cool and add half a dessertspoon of cider vinegar. Gargle every four hours.

Tinctures to make a more sophisticated mixture can be purchased from a herbal supplier.

Tinctures of:
  Golden seal (*Hydrastis canadensis*) 5 ml
  Balm of gilead (*Populus gileadensis*) 5 ml
  Myrrh (*Commiphora molmol*) 5 ml
  Liquorice (*Glycyrrhiza glabra*) 5 ml
  Oil of cinnamon 4 drops

Add water to 200 ml. Shake well before use and use a teaspoon of this mixture in a cup of warm water as a gargle.

Commercial preparation

Weleda's gargle and mouthwash.

Any sore throat or hoarseness which lasts more than a few days should be examined by a specialist.

Coughs

If a cold goes to the chest or an infection of the bronchial tubes occurs directly, a cough will certainly result. This is a natural reflex (the vital force is at work) to clear the airways of mucus produced by the cells lining the respiratory tract, which immobilizes bacteria and protects the airways from damage. For this reason it is unwise to suppress a cough. Many herbal remedies help the natural process of expectoration.

A simple kitchen remedy:

> Large onion
> Honey

Slice the onion into rings and place in a fairly deep bowl. Cover the rings with organic honey and leave for eight hours. Strain off the juice of the onion, which is now mixed with the honey. Take this honey elixir in dessertspoon doses every two to four hours.

A general cough remedy:

> 2 woody liquorice sticks (*Glycyrrhiza glabra*)
> Marshmallow root (*Althaea officinalis*) 8 gm
> Wild cherry bark (*Prunus serotina*) 8 gm
> Coltsfoot flowers (*Tussilago farfara*) 8 gm
> Borage leaves and flowers (*Borago officinalis*) 8 gm
> Hyssop (*Hyssopus officinalis*) 8 gm
> Linseed (whole seed) (*Linum usitatissimum*) 30 gm
> Juice of half a lemon

On to the ingredients pour $1\frac{1}{4}$ litres boiling water. Stir well and cover. Let it stand for an hour. Re-heat and strain. Drink a hot cupful, sweetened with organic honey, every two hours.

Rub the chest with camphorated oil or Olbas oil diluted with a little vegetable oil.

Eat garlic, onions, ginger, cabbage and sweet almonds. Avoid mucus-forming foods. If you smoke, give it up!

Note: Herbal practitioners will vary their remedies to treat several different kinds of cough. Any cough that lasts more than a few days must be diagnosed and treated by a professional. It can be a sign of serious disease.

Styes

A stye is an inflammation of the small glands, which secrete a lubricating fluid, located at the base of the eyelashes. Such infections may be a sign that the sufferer is run down and needs to look at his or her general health.

Create a lint compress of fresh, preferably organically grown, parsley, or marigold flower petals. Using distilled water, either blanch the extract or steam it over a boiling pan. Place it on to the lint and, while it is still warm, apply it to the stye, so that the parsley or marigold petals come into direct contact with the infection.

Tired and sore eyes

Take a cucumber from the fridge. Slice it and lie quietly with a slice over each closed eye. This is good for tired eyes.

Make an infusion by placing a tea-bag of fennel or chamomile (*Matricaria chamomilla*) in a cup of boiling water, or use one teaspoon of eyebright (*Euphrasia officinalis*) to a cup of boiling water. Strain, allow to cool and bathe the eye, taking care to sterilize the eye-bath before use, and not to use the same infusion-water for both eyes.

A good general eye-lotion can be made up as follows:

> Eyebright tincture (*Euphrasia officinalis*) 2 ml
> Golden seal tincture (*Hydrastis canadensis*) 1 ml
> Rosewater 97 ml

Bathe the eyes as above.

Cuts

Any serious cut should be taken to the doctor. Bathe minor ones with diluted marigold flower (*Calendula officinalis*) tincture. You can make this yourself by macerating as many marigold flower heads as you can get, in half a litre of vodka. Leave for a month, shaking regularly, and then express all the liquid through a muslin bag. Keep in a dark glass bottle for emergencies. This is a good remedy for shaving cuts, too.

Scar tissue can be helped to heal by using a mixture of comfrey ointment and Vitamin E oil. This is available commercially, but you can also blend the two together yourself.

Bruises and sprains

If you bruise easily you may be short of Vitamin C, which can be taken together with rutin tablets.

Bruises and sprains respond well to compresses of witch hazel (*Hamamelis virginiana*), comfrey (*Symphytum officinale*) – ointment or oil of comfrey can also be used – and arnica (*Arnica montana*).

Dilute 2.5 ml of arnica tincture in 250 ml of water, and bathe the bruise or sprained area. Daisies (*Bellis perennis*) belong to the same family as arnica, and may also be used as a compress for bruises. Their old name was bruisewort.

Ice-packs are also useful, and witch hazel (*Hamamelis virginiana*) can actually be poured into an ice-tray and frozen before use, so combining these two therapies. If you have nothing else, bind a cabbage leaf over any bruised or painful area.

Burns

The best first-aid for a burn is cold water. Afterwards there are several herbal remedies that can bring relief from pain and promote healing.

Apply some lavender oil to the burnt area, or you can use comfrey ointment. Also useful is St John's wort (*Hypericum perforatum*) oil. This oil is made by macerating the flowers and leaves of St John's wort in olive or sunflower oil, for a

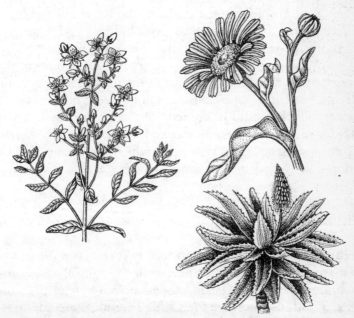

St John's wort, Garden marigold, Aloe vera

month or more, in a sunny place. The vegetable oil will become blood-red as the oil contained in the plant is released. Strain off the oil and keep it in a dark glass bottle. (This oil is also excellent for neuralgia and spinal nerve pain, gently massaged into the painful area.)

Lastly, but by no means least, every house should have an *Aloe vera* plant, which is easy to grow indoors. Break off one of its leaves and immediately a copious flow of mucilage is released, which is superb for healing and cooling burnt skin.

Shock

Many herbalists make good use of the flower essences, the Bach Flower Remedies, which are used to treat psychological problems. One of them, the Rescue Remedy, is excellent for treating shock in both humans and animals.

If the patient is unconscious, the remedy can still be used by rubbing a drop or two on to the pulse points at the wrist, or by moistening the lips of the unconscious person. If the patient is conscious, put four drops in a glass of water, which should be sipped. The same remedy is available in cream form too. Someone in shock may also benefit from sipping a glass of water into which has been mixed no more than five drops of arnica tincture.

Stings

Extract a bee sting using sterilized tweezers (run the end of the tweezers through a flame); wash the painful area using sodium bicarbonate (baking soda) applied as a paste to the site. Wasps do not leave their sting behind. Wasp and mosquito bites can be treated by applying lemon juice, witch hazel or cider vinegar to the sting or bite. Alternatively, apply crushed plantain leaves or a sliced onion to the affected area. Lavender oil, too, can be soothing.

Insects can be repelled by rubbing one's skin with citronella, lavender or tea-tree oil, all diluted with a little olive oil or alcohol.

Nosebleed

The old English name for yarrow (*Achillea millefolium*) is 'nosebleed'. Crush a leaf of yarrow and push it gently up the affected nostril. Be careful not to push the leaf too far up the nostril in children. Apply a cold compress to the back of the neck.

Chilblains

Mix powdered cayenne pepper (*Capsicum minimum*) with talcum powder and put this in your socks. Use hot foot baths of ginger (30 gm) and cinnamon (two sticks) to a litre of water. To this add 250 gm of magnesium sulphate (Epsom salt) crystals. Bathe the feet daily. The water can be retained and used again for four or five days.

Travel sickness

A three-year study recently completed at Vermont University in the United States showed that chewing a bit of ginger just before setting out on a journey is as good as any equivalent drug treatment. A drink of ginger is said to have been used by the pirate Sir Henry Morgan to dose his crew against sea-sickness. No doubt in true piratical style they combined it with rum!

Indigestion

Regular bouts of indigestion need investigating. An adjustment of diet or mode of eating can often do much to solve the problem. It is a mistake to take antacids because the natural state of the stomach is acid, so that the alkaline antacids, in the long term, merely provoke the stomach to produce even more acid. If you have indigestion try the following tea:

> Gentian root (*Gentiana lutea*) 8 gm
> Angelica root (*Angelica archangelica*) 8 gm
> Anise (*Pimpinella anisum*) 15 gm
> Peppermint (*Mentha piperita*) 15 gm
> Chamomile (*Matricaria chamomilla*) 15 gm
> Dried mandarin peel (*Citrus reticulata*) 4 pieces
> Liquorice (*Glycyrrhiza glabra*) 1 stick broken and crushed

Put the liquorice stick, gentian and angelica root in 1 litre of water. Bring it to the boil and simmer for ten minutes. Take it off the heat and add the rest of the ingredients. Cover and let it stand for ten minutes before straining. Drink a hot cupful of this tea after eating.

Also useful are slippery elm pills (*Ulmus fulva*), which are available commercially.

For acid digestion take 1–2 vegetable charcoal tablets after eating. Weak meadowsweet (*Filipendula ulmaria*) tea is also beneficial.

Diarrhoea

Acute diarrhoea may occur when the digestive system tries to rid itself of some toxin or disagreeable food. Diarrhoea may signal serious disease, so if continuous for more than a day or two, or if it persistently recurs, professional help be sought. Diarrhoea in young children (like vomiting) can quickly lead to dehydration and the loss of electrolytes, with serious consequences. Parents must not delay proper treatment of any child with more than a mild bout of diarrhoea.

Harmful substances in the bowel can be neutralized using absorbants like pectin, found in raw apples, and the tannins of astringent herbs, which help restore the tone and the function of the large bowel. Eat plenty of garlic for its antibiotic action.

To control diarrhoea:

> Tormentil (*Potentilla tormentilla*) 30 gm
> Cinnamon 1 stick, broken
> Caraway seeds 1 tsp
> Ginger 2 slices

Add the ingredients to 600 ml water, bring to the boil and simmer for fifteen minutes. Strain and drink a wine glassful four times a day.

Powdered rhubarb root (*Rheum officinale*) is a herbal remedy that has a dual activity. In large doses it is a laxative but in doses of about half a gram (fifteen grains) it can effectively stop a bout of diarrhoea. Half a gram of the powdered root can be mixed with honey or put into a size oo capsule. Take this dose three times a day.

After the acute episode is controlled, mix:

> Arrowroot powder (*Maranta arundinaceae*) 8 gm
> Slippery elm powder (*Ulmus fulva*) 8 gm
> Cinnamon powder 1 pinch

Blend a teaspoon of this into a little plain yoghurt and take this throughout the day. Also eat stewed apple and cinnamon.

To restore electrolyte balance and fluids in both adults and children, drink warm water sweetened with organic honey.

Insomnia

Many herbs encourage relaxation of the muscles and nervous system.

Teas of the following can help the insomniac and are non-addictive:

> Limeflower (*Tilia europaea*)
> Chamomile (*Matricaria chamomilla*)
> Passion flower (*Passiflora incarnata*)
> Valerian (*Valeriana officinalis*)
> Hops (*Humulus lupulus*)

A teaspoon of cider vinegar and honey taken in a cup of hot water before bedtime can be helpful, as can soaking in a hot bath with a few drops of lavender oil. Alternatively make a strong infusion of limeflowers with 30 gm of herb to 500 ml of boiling water. Strain and pour this into the bath.

Sesame seeds and sesame paste (tahini) are rich in calcium and can be eaten to strengthen the nervous system. Oats are also food for the nervous system, while lettuce helps the nervous system to relax. Hop pillows can help too.

Avoid caffeinated drinks; meditate to avoid stress and anxiety.

CHAPTER SIX

CHEMISTRY

This chapter is about the chemistry of plants. In some ways it follows on from the last part of Chapter 2 in which I discussed the modern scientific approach to herbal medicine. The modern herbalist has access to an enormous amount of scientific data about plant medicines, hitherto unavailable. This valuable information can undoubtedly increase the herbalist's understanding and skill, for the chemical analysis of plants has revealed myriad substances which have evident effect on the body and mind. An old Chinese saying however warns that 'the finger pointing at the moon is not the moon'. In the final analysis it is not the isolated chemicals which are responsible for the healing action of a plant, but the whole plant itself. The chemical constituents of plants are only indications of their possible use; we should not allow them to obscure our overall view. Each chemical component is like a single instrument in the orchestral harmony that is the whole plant. With this in mind let us look at some of the most important plant chemicals.

Alkaloids

The function of alkaloids was also debated in Chapter 2. All alkaloids contain nitrogen; this is their chemical signature. They were given their name by the first scientists to discover them, who saw them as plant alkalis. The names of several specific alkaloids, like nicotine, caffeine and morphine, could not be more familiar to us. Alkaloids usually have a very bitter taste and, as mentioned earlier, a potent physiological effect on human beings, influencing the central nervous system in particular. Many plants contain several alkaloids. The opium poppy, from which the first alkaloid, narcotine, was isolated in 1803, contains about thirty other alkaloids, including morphine and codeine.

Alkaloid levels in plants can vary considerably depending on the time of year, or even the time of day. Generally speaking, they attain their highest concentration immediately before or at the beginning of the flowering phase. The discovery of alkaloids in many famous healing plants has helped to explain how they work. But the complex interaction of several alkaloids, to say nothing of the other components of plants, will give quite different effects to that gained from a single isolated alkaloid (see the discussion in Chapter 2).

Tannins

As the name suggests, tannin is used to tan leather. Oak bark, which has a high tannin content, was usually used for this process. The tannin it contains coagulates the protein in animal hides, rendering them impervious to putrefaction, converting them to leather. Tannin, extracted from oak galls, was also used to make ink. Iron salts were added to the solution of tannin extract, giving the ink a characteristic blue colour. Today, as home wine-makers will know, tannin is used to clarify wine due to its ability to combine with and precipitate proteins and allied nitrogenous substances, which tend to cause wine-hazes.

Tannins are also useful to the plants which contain them. They occur widely throughout the plant kingdom (especially in the Rosaceae, Ericaceae, Salicaceae and Leguminosae families) and are usually concentrated in the outer part of the plant, like the bark, where their coagulating action on protein wards off would-be predators.

In medicine, tannin is important because of its astringent action. Astringent herbs like witch hazel, rich in tannins, cause a thin layer to form on wounds or inflamed mucous membranes, so promoting rapid healing. Herbs containing tannin are therefore used externally to treat minor burns, cuts, inflammations, swellings, haemorrhoids and varicose ulcers. Taken internally they are useful in controlling diarrhoea (see the mention of tormentil in Chapter 5), healing peptic ulcers and reducing catarrhal secretions in colitis. Once exposed to air, tannins undergo chemical changes, and so plants containing them will lose their effectiveness if stored for too long.

Cardiac glycosides

These are present in some well-known European plants such as foxglove (*Digitalis*), squills (*Urginea maritima*), lily of the valley (*Convallaria majalis*), pheasant's eye (*Adonis vernalis*) and wallflowers (*Cheiranthus cheiri*). Further afield they are found in the seeds of the Strophanthus species of plants, some thirty types of which are indigenous to East and West Africa, where an extract of the seeds, which contain the glycoside ouabain, was used to make arrow poisons. Cardiac glycosides are a combination of a sugar with a non-sugar. The latter is the more physiologically active part, although the sugar helps the uptake of the glycoside by the heart. This is another example of the importance of the apparently less active constituents in natural remedies.

Cardiac glycosides have an extraordinary capacity to support a weakened or failing heart; they increase its muscle power without causing a corresponding increase in oxygen demand. Orthodox medicine generally uses the cardiac glycosides extracted from the foxglove, but herbalists prefer to use lily of the valley because its cardiac glycosides are released more slowly than those of the foxglove, and they are more easily excreted by the body too, so avoiding a toxic accumulation.

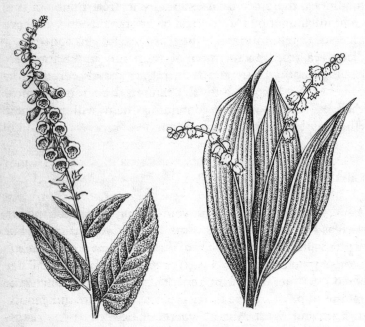

Foxglove, Lily of the valley

Saponins

Saponins are another type of glycoside. They derive their name from their ability to dissolve in water to form a lather. Soapwort (*Saponaria officinalis*), a plant rich in saponins, was used to manufacture soap. The lather that plants like soapwort produce is an emulsion, which lifts dirt and grease off the skin.

Saponins are poisonous when injected directly into the bloodstream, where they cause mayhem by breaking down red blood cells – a process called haemolysis. Taken orally however they are hardly absorbed at all. Indeed, some familiar herbs and vegetables like asparagus, oats, tomatoes, spinach and haricot beans contain saponins which assist in digestion. Saponins can actually help the body to absorb calcium and silicon.

Several plants, like cowslip roots (*Primula veris*), mullein (*Verbascum thapsus*), liquorice (*Glycyrrhiza glabra*) and sweet violet (*Viola odorata*), have an expectorant action, probably derived from the irritation of nerve ends in the digestive tract by the saponins they contain. Stimulation of these nerves in the gut wall causes reflex coughing. The diuretic effect of other herbs like cornsilk (*Zea mays*) may be due to their saponins.

But the most fascinating aspect of saponins lies in their structural similarity to human sex and stress hormones, secreted by the ovaries, testes and adrenal glands. The steroidal or hormone-like saponins resemble cholesterol, cortisone, oestrogen, progesterone and Vitamin D. They are to be found in members of the lily family, like the trillium and sarsaparilla species; in the wild yam family; and the Solanaceae family, for example – in woody night-shade (*Solanum dulcamara*). Closely related to these steroidal saponins are the other kind of plant saponins – the triterpenoids. These are present in the famous oriental plant ginseng (*Panax ginseng*), and its allied species. Ginseng has a demonstrable ability to regulate the human hormone balance and counter the effect of stress. This harmonizing action is termed an *adaptogenic* effect.

Many other herbs containing saponins also display this hormone-regulating action – for example, blue cohosh

(*Caulophyllum thalictroides*), black cohosh (*Cimicifuga racemosa*), false unicorn root (*Chamaelirium luteum*) and members of the sarsaparilla species. Several herbs containing saponins, like horse chestnut (*Aesculus hippocastanum*), liquorice and wild yam (*Dioscorea villosa*), have an anti-inflammatory action.

The close association between plant saponins and human hormones was exploited by the brilliant and eccentric scientist Russell Marker. In 1943 he astonished the world when, on a shoestring budget in a makeshift laboratory in Mexico City, he made two kilos of pure progesterone from the Mexican wild yam (*Dioscorea mexicana*). Just nine years earlier another scientist had triumphantly produced twenty milligrams of progesterone from the ovaries of 50,000 sows! Marker's discovery made him a rich man, for the market price of pure progesterone was then $80 per gram. Until 1970 the steroidal saponin disogenin, extracted from the Mexican yam, was the sole source of the hormonal material for the manufacture of the contraceptive pill.

Anthraquinones

Anthraquinones are also glycosides and are plant dyes. They are found in dyer's madder (*Rubia tinctorum*), which was used to produce commercial dyes. The anthraquinone glycosides irritate the large bowel and so have a laxative effect. Plants containing anthraquinones, like senna, cascara, rhubarb, alder, buckthorn and aloes, should not be habitually used, since the bowel will become reliant on them and normal evacuation will not occur. I well remember attending a post-mortem of a man who used senna for several years (this was not the cause of death). His bowel told the story, for it was dyed a bright orange!

Flavonoids

Flavonoids also often appear in plants as glycosides, but may be in their free state too. They are found especially in plants of the Polygonacea, Rutaceae, Leguminosae, Umbelliferae and Compositae families. Like anth-raquinones, they have also been used as dyes and give many flowers such as cowslip their yellow colour (the Latin word *flavus* means yellow). Flavonoid-containing plants like buchu (*Agathosma betulina*) and broom (*Sarothamnus scoparius*) are diuretic, while others like liquorice (*Glycyrrhiza glabra*) and parsley are anti-spasmodic. In recent years the importance of the bio-flavonoids, like rutin and hesperidin, (formerly called Vitamin P) has been emphasized. They are invariably found in Vitamin C-rich plants and act in the body synergistically with Vitamin C, increasing its bio-availability i.e. the ability of the body to make use of it. Bio-flavonoids strengthen the capillary walls, and so are useful in treating bruising and bleeding, such as post-natal bleeding and nose-bleeding. They have anti-bacterial and anti-viral properties, and rutin is also used to treat high blood pressure.

Essential oils

Essential oils are volatile substances easily released from plants, especially when their leaves are crushed or they are warmed by the sun. The oils have a rich aromatic smell, as in peppermint (main oil, menthol), thyme (main oil, thymol) and sage (main oil, thujone). Many aromatic plants contain a score or more of these oils, subtly blended to give each plant its characteristic smell. In some plants, like conifers, these oils oxidize to produce resins and gums.

Volatile oils have a wide range of actions since, as their name implies, they permeate easily throughout the body. Their molecules can affect the brain directly through the nose. The smell of mint or rosemary, for instance, can increase awareness and concentration. Taken internally as part of the whole plant * these oils are mildly irritant on the mucous membranes of the mouth, imparting a feeling of warmth and increasing salivation, so aiding digestion. Their irritant effect tends to cause a quickening of breathing and stimulates the heart and circulation. These oils are excreted through the lungs, kidneys and skin, so that they can act as expectorants, diuretics and diaphoretics. Volatile oils have an antibiotic action too. The germicidal properties of many oils, like thymol from thyme or allicin from garlic, have been scientifically endorsed. Some essential oils are anthelmintic (expelling worms). Taken after meals as a tea, plants like mint or fennel can relax the digestive tract and relieve indigestion and flatulence. They also help to counter the griping pains of purgatives.

Plants containing volatile oils tend to lose these oils easily and so when preparing them for drinking they should not be boiled. Moreover, once the tisane is made, the pot or cup should be covered to prevent the steam carrying off the precious aromatic content.

If volatile oils are inhaled in steam they make viscous, mucous secretions more fluid, and so help to relieve congestion in the chest, nose and sinuses.

When applied externally many volatile oils have a numbing, anaesthetic effect. Clove-oil is used to ease toothache. Some more powerful oils, like mustard oil, are used for their rubefacient and irritant effect in anti-rheumatic liniments. Care has to be taken to avoid blistering.

---

* Some extracted, pure volatile oils can be taken internally in tiny amounts. This should only be done under professional supervision, since these oils are very powerful.

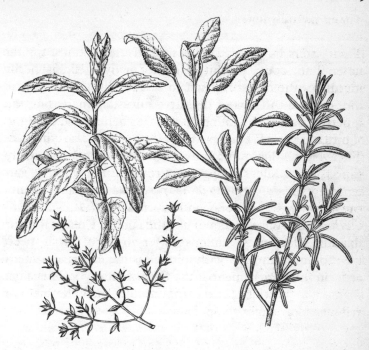

Mint, Sage, Thyme, Rosemary

Lastly, many essential oils are important in flavouring food. They enhance taste and digestion.

Vegetable oils

Vegetable oils are also called fixed oils, to distinguish them from volatile oils. Unlike animal fats, they are mostly unsaturated. Saturated oils and fats can contribute to high cholesterol levels. Cholesterol is a major constituent of the plaque of fat (atheroma) that thickens the wall of blood vessels, and which predisposes an individual to conditions like heart disease and strokes.

Bitter principles

Plant bitters have a wide chemical diversity, but a similar action in the body. The bitter taste of many medicinal herbs stimulates the digestive tract to secrete digestive enzymes and increase the flow of digestive juices, so increasing the appetite. This is the rationale that lies behind the drinking of bitter apperitifs before a meal. Bitter tastes also stimulate the liver, further improving digestion. There are many famous bitter tonics, like gentian root (*Gentiana lutea*), and centaury (*Centaurium erythraea*). All the Artemisia family are also rich in bitters, and wormwood (*Artemisia absinthium*) was once used to make the famous French liqueur absinthe. The most famous bitter drink of all is beer, brewed for centuries with bitter-tasting hops, despite a petition from Parliament at the time of Henry VIII against the hop as 'a wicked weed that would spoil the taste of drink and endanger the people'.

Mucilages

Mucilages are the slimy, stringy exudates from many plants. These comprise long chains of sugars (polysaccharides), which swell in water, forming a soothing gel. Mucilage tends to retain heat and so plants which contain mucilage are often used externally as hot compresses to draw boils and abscesses.

Internally, mucilage has a healing and soothing action on damaged mucous membranes lining the digestive tract. It seems that mucilage can also soothe by reflex, via the nerves in the gut wall and through the spinal nerves, other parts of the body related embryologically to the digestive tract, such as the lungs and urinary tract. Typical plants containing mucilage are marshmallow (*Althaea officinalis*), comfrey

(*Symphytum officinale*), linseed (*Linum usitatissimum*), psyllium seed (*Plantago psyllium*) and Irish moss (*Chondrus crispus*). The linseeds and psyllium seeds swell with water, making an effective yet gentle bulk laxative.

Organic acids

Organic acids are found throughout the plant kingdom, where they participate in essential metabolism. Acids, like malic, citric and tartaric acid, are most concentrated in unripe fruits. Such acids tend to give even ripe fruit their refreshing quality. Vitamin C is ascorbic acid, and is widely found in herbs, fruits and vegetables. Citric and tartaric acid are anti-bacterial and stimulate the flow of saliva. For this reason an apple a day may at least keep the dentist away. These acids are mildly laxative and diuretic. A large number of other acids exist in the plant world, including salicylic acid, mentioned in Chapter 2.

One particular type of plant acid may not be good for some people. This is oxalic acid found in the leaves of rhubarb and sorrel. These sharp little crystals can trigger off an attack of gout or kidney stones in the susceptible.

Vitamins and trace elements

With the exception of Vitamin D, plants, fruit and vegetables supply the complete range of vitamins. Vitamin A is not found in its pure form, but occurs as provitamin A (beta-carotene), which has a yellow pigment. This is transformed in the liver to Vitamin A. Nature supplies a balance of herbs and minerals, making plants an ideal way to obtain these vital ingredients. An example is the number of Vitamin C-rich vegetables and fruit, like dandelion, watercress, nettles and rosehips, which are also rich in iron. Iron is much better absorbed in the presence of Vitamin C. Dandelion is also rich in potassium, which makes it an ideal diuretic (hence its French name *pissenlit*) because, unlike its drug counterparts, it does not leach potassium from the body. Seaweeds, like kelp, and plants, like alfalfa, are other fine sources of trace elements.

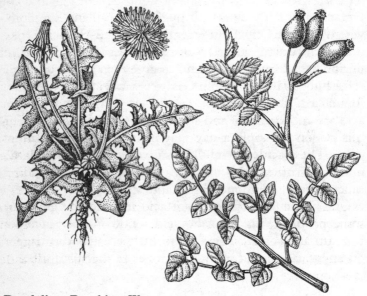

Dandelion, Rosehips, Watercress

CHAPTER SEVEN

PREPARATIONS

One of the great pleasures of being a herbalist is collecting or growing herbs. An early-morning expedition into the woods and fields to gather medicinal plants is a marvellously peaceful and rejuvenating way to start the day. Growing herbs is also a rewarding activity, and is a subject in itself. If you want to know more about this, consult one of the books recommended in the reading list at the end of this book.

Some people talk to their plants because they say it helps the plants to grow. Whether you believe this or not, I think the spirit in which one collects herbs is important. We should have a care for the herbs and roots we use, and give thanks for their existence. Plants connect with and store the earth-energy at the place where they grow, and can transmit this to someone who is sick. It was for this reason that the herbalists of old prohibited the use of iron implements to cut herbs; iron was thought to damage this subtle healing force.

Apart from acknowledging a debt to nature, one is required by law to ask permission of the landowner before collecting herbs. Certain rare species are protected and may not be picked or uprooted in any circumstances.

In the old days people believed that the *time* when herbs were collected was important, and would affect their potency. Their medicinal properties were seen to wax and wane with the moon, the seasons, and even during the day. St John's wort was so christened because it was believed that the plant should be gathered on or about St John's day (midsummer's day) to obtain its maximum effect. In fact, this was good advice; this is the time when the plant comes into flower, and so is the best time to harvest it.

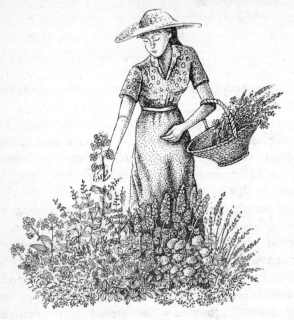

According to French herbal tradition herbs and flowers should not be collected at full moon because the moon saps their strength. Roots, on the other hand, were held to be at their most potent just before full moon. A Tibetan herbal doctor told me how in Tibet some plants were traditionally harvested by moonlight, whilst others were collected during the day. Until recently science scoffed at these 'superstitions', but discoveries about plant and animal biorhythms have made us think twice. Scientists have discovered that the morphine content of the opium poppy capsule is higher at 11 a.m. than at 3 p.m., and is at its greatest concentration for around three weeks after flowering. In winter, rhubarb root contains virtually no anthraquinone, which usually gives it its laxative property, but the plant manufactures this active principle when warmer weather comes.

Generally speaking, leaves should be gathered when the flowers are beginning to open. Any that are mottled or damaged must be discarded. Flowers are at their best just before they are fully expanded, and underground parts of a plant should be collected as the aerial parts die down. Bark can be gathered in the spring as the sap rises; care should be taken not to damage the tree by over-collection. We do most of our collecting on warm days just after the sun has dried up any overnight dew or rain. Barks, however, are best collected after a period of damp weather since then they separate most easily from the tree. Gums and resins are collected after hot, dry weather.

Roots and rhizomes must be shaken well to free them from the soil. Shaking or brushing roots may be sufficient to dislodge sandy soil, but if uprooted from clay soil the roots will probably need a good wash. Before drying, any worm-eaten or diseased roots should be discarded. The good roots can then be cut up ready for drying.

Make sure that you do not overpick any area, leaving plenty of what you are collecting behind to propagate in the coming years. Gather your plants well away from towns and roads. Lead used as an anti-knock agent in petrol is sprayed over hedgerows and fields by passing cars, where plants will absorb considerable quantities of it. Chemical fertilizers, herbicides, insecticides and pesticides sprayed over crops will invalidate the medicinal qualities of plants in the vicinity. The sixteenth-century London herbalist, John Gerard, wrote that he collected some of his plants from the ditches of Piccadilly and the marshes of Paddington in central London. In this respect, how much easier it was to be a herbalist in his day! Today's herbalists have to range far and wide to find uncontaminated plants. Many herbalists buy their herbal medicines from reputable suppliers, a list of whom you can find in the resource section at the end of this book. This is particularly recommended if you are not good at recognizing plants. Plants are sometimes confused, with disastrous consequences. For example, foxglove has been confused with mullein, and the poisonous hemlock with wild carrot.

Put the herbs you gather in wicker baskets or paper bags. Never use plastic. On a warm summer's day, fermentation will begin quickly so plants must be spread out to dry as soon as possible. Drying herbs in one's house can cause problems. I well remember the swarm of insects I released into my rooms when I dried a particular batch of marigold flowers. A dry, well-ventilated outhouse is ideal. To ensure effective drying it is important to allow air to circulate around the herbs. Small bundles of plants can be hung from the ceiling, or a series of wooden racks can be used, allowing at least 15 cm (6 inches) between the stacked trays. As herbs dry they should be moved downwards, so that the more moist herbs are always at the top of the stack. This prevents drier herbs from becoming damp again. Label each hanging bunch or tray with the name of the herb being dried. Once herbs are dry they are often much more difficult to recognize. Be careful not to spread herbs on the racks too thickly. Herbs should not be dried in direct sunlight since valuable components like volatile oils will vapourize and disappear. Herbs, leaves and flowers can be dried in a temperature of 20–40 °C. Barks and roots can stand somewhat higher temperatures, of 30–40 °C. You can tell when your plants are dry because they should fracture but not crumble. They should retain their colour and aroma.

Similar care needs to be taken when storing herbs. Because of the bleaching effect of sunlight, herbs should be stored in a dark place, either in paper bags, cardboard boxes (shoe boxes are ideal because they can be stacked), or glass bottles with air-tight lids. Again, plastic bags must not be used. Always label your stock with the name of the plant and the date when it was harvested. Ideally aerial parts of the plant should not be kept for more than a year (old herbs make excellent compost), while roots and bark may generally be kept for two years. Examine your stock at regular intervals to check that there is no mildew or infestation.

Herbs can be prescribed in many different ways. The manner of prescription is often as important in therapeutic terms as the herbs that are used. Different methods of processing the same herb will extract different ingredients. For example, alcohol will extract oils, gums and resins more readily than water or glycerol.

Infusions and decoctions

Infusions are made by pouring boiling water over dried or fresh herbs. Water is an excellent solvent, extracting gums, mucilages, saponins and tannins, but, as mentioned, is not so effective when it comes to oils. Spring water or filtered water is preferable to ordinary tap water. The infusion pot or cup should be covered to prevent volatile oils being dissipated in the steam.

Decoctions are made by boiling in water harder plant substances, such as roots or bark. Roots and barks containing volatile oils, like valerian root, should only be boiled for a short time, and left to steep in the water as they cool. Never use aluminium cooking utensils for making up herbal medicines, since minute amounts of aluminium could enter your preparations. Use enamel, reinforced glass, or stainless-steel saucepans instead.

The traditional proportion for an infusion is 30 gm of dried herb to 500 ml of water. Infuse this for fifteen minutes before drinking it. For a decoction use 600 ml of water to

30 gm of dried root or bark. This should be brought to the boil and simmered for fifteen to twenty minutes. The dose for both infusions and decoctions is a wineglassful, three times daily. Keep any fluid left over in the fridge for no more than twenty-four hours. Re-heat (but do not boil) before taking this. This dosage is good for acute disease.

Chronic diseases, in my experience, require less strong brews. I usually recommend two or three teaspoons of dried plant material to a cup of boiling water. A similarly weaker decoction can be made by putting three or four teaspoons of dried and cut roots or bark in three cups of water, and simmering them for fifteen minutes before drinking. When making a preparation containing roots, bark and herb, decoct the hard substances first and then pour the strained boiling water on to the herb. Leave this to infuse for fifteen minutes as usual.

Cultural conditioning often determines the strength and kind of herbal preparation that patients consider acceptable. In China strong decoctions (*tang*, literally 'soups') are the rule, made with about 50 gm of dried herbs, which is a daily dose. Most western patients would gag on this invariably bitter-tasting brew. In any case, a gentle prescription often gets good results.

In the West, infusions and decoctions may be taken on an empty stomach, so long as the digestive system is up to it. They are prescribed to be taken just before meals if the intention is to stimulate gastric juices. Chinese herbal tradition offers a somewhat more intricate approach to the timing of taking herbal medicine. As in the West, herbs are taken after meals if the digestion is weak. Tonic herbs, however, which treat general weakness, are usually taken before meals. Herbs which treat the bones and marrow are thought to be best taken at night. They should be taken after meals if they are for diseases of the chest and above, but before meals if the disease is below the chest. Both the Chinese

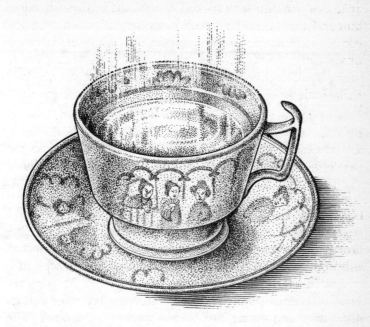

The infusion cup

and western systems agree that medicine to expel worms should be taken on an empty stomach.

All systems of herbal medicine use weaker dosages for old people and children. One rule of thumb uses Cowling's formula, which divides the patient's next birthday by twenty-four. So to obtain the dose for a child of three you would need to divide four by twenty-four, indicating that the child would need one sixth of the adult dose.

Although infusions and decoctions are thought less potent than alcoholic extracts, in my experience they are the best way to treat acute disease. In the discussion of the treatment of fevers (see Chapter 3) we saw how hot infusions help to bring about therapeutic sweating. The famous physiomedicalist Doctor Thurston, writing in 1897, was a firm advocate of infusions and decoctions in these circum-stances.

While the writer is not the champion of a retrograde return to the crude methods of the 'tea doctors', as our early practitioners were dubbed, he does advocate the use of infusions and decoc-tions in all severe cases . . . For we are sure that by using attractive forms of infusion cups, nicely decorated and artistically shaped, and in this way utilizing the modern tendency to fads, the hand-painted China infusion cup would do much to popularize and again bring into general use this most effective of preparations.[1]

Tinctures

Tinctures are made by extracting the medicinal properties of herbs by macerating them for at least two weeks in a precise mixture of water and alcohol. While, as we have seen, water extracts many of the vital constituents of plants, oils, gums and resins are best extracted in alcohol. The alcohol also preserves the tincture, which is usually ex-pressed from the herb by use of a press. Tinctures may also be made by percolation; a continuous flow of a mixture of water and alcohol filters through the powdered herb and is collected at the bottom of the percolation chamber.

Most tinctures are made by macerating 200 gm of dried herb in a litre of a mixture of water and alcohol. The strength of the alcohol is determined by what has to be extracted from the particular herb. It may vary from that of a fortified wine at twenty-five per cent to the strongest Polish vodka at ninety per cent. Lower alcoholic strengths are always used where possible.

Although amongst herbalists in the UK tinctures are the most popular way to prescribe herbs, they are not always suitable to treat every condition. According to the Chinese, alcohol is hot, pungent, sweet and ascending. It is yang in nature, stimulating both the Qi (vital force) and blood, unblocking the meridians or energy channels, and reinforcing the actions of the herbs with which it is combined. It is ideally suited to treating deficiency diseases, where the body energy is reduced or weak, and is also particularly good for treating arthritis, caused by exposure to wind, damp and cold (a common problem in this country!). On the other hand, alcohol is not recommended for those suffering from full, fiery or hot diseases, where there may be a high fever and a bounding pulse. It is also wise for a patient to avoid taking alcohol if there is a problem with liver disease, and of course it is contra-indicated if the patient is an alcoholic.

To make tinctures at home you can use vodka or brandy, which are about forty per cent alcohol (seventy per cent proof). A cheap wine press and muslin or nylon bags can be used to express the tincture after the maceration period. The usual dose of tincture is one teaspoon three times a day, usually taken after meals.

Glycerol

Glycerol can also be used to preserve an aqueous extract of a plant. This is especially useful for mucilaginous roots, like those of comfrey and marshmallow. Place 200 gm of the dried herb in a saucepan and add a litre of water. Bring this to the boil and reduce the volume to about 600 ml. Leave the root to macerate in the water for four hours before straining and pressing. To the 600 ml add 400 ml of glycerol, and use exactly as a tincture (see above). Aerial parts of the plant can be extracted by putting 200 gm of herb in a pot and pouring on 600 ml of boiling water. Cover and leave overnight to macerate; proceed as previously.

Most commercial glycerol is of animal origin. Suppliers of the more expensive plant glycerol only sell in bulk.

Fluid extracts

Fluid extracts are also known as liquid extracts and have been the most commonly produced commercial herb extracts. They are highly concentrated preparations where one part by volume of the liquid extract represents one part by weight of the herb – that is, a litre of fluid extract represents a kilogram of herb. There are several different techniques to accomplish this. One process uses extraction by alcohol which is then evaporated off the solid extract in a vacuum. This solid extract is then dissolved to the required strength in diluted alcohol. A cold percolation technique, which does not damage delicate plant constituents by heat, is now increasingly being used.

Syrups

Because many people eat too much sugar, diabetes and its opposite condition, hypoglycaemia (low blood sugar), are on the increase. If you suffer from either of these conditions, syrups are not for you. Syrups should be made with honey rather than sugar. Honey is rich in trace elements and also often contains some vitamins. It is a natural antibiotic, and helps expectoration too. It is an ideal medium for preparing cough medicines, and obviously is popular with most children. In China, where people do not eat vast amounts of sugar, syrups are considered especially beneficial for the treatment of chronic debilitating diseases and (as in the West) for coughs and sore throats.

A syrup can be made by decocting herbs in a litre of

water. When it has cooled, strain it and weigh it. Add to this a quarter of its weight of honey. Heat the liquid gently, stirring it until it thickens. As when making jam, skim off any scum that forms on the surface. The taste of bitter herbs can further be disguised by the addition of liquorice, mint or aniseed as flavouring agents. The dose of syrup taken will, to some extent, depend upon what is in it, but often a dessertspoon is taken three or four times a day.

Powders

Many herbs can be powdered using a coffee grinder. Some herbs can be purchased as powders, which saves a lot of trouble. These powders can either be mixed with honey to make an electuary (sugar-free jams are an alternative to honey), or put into gelatine capsules. There are two main sizes of capsules suited to taking herb powders, the 0 and larger 00 size. Size 0 capsules will hold around 350 gm of powdered herb, so that around nine of these capsules are required a day (three, three times a day) to get a minimum adult dose. Size 00 capsules will take about 500 gm of powdered herb, so to achieve a similar dose six have to be taken a day. Making up a large number of capsules by hand is a fiddly and time-consuming business. The address of where to obtain simple and relatively inexpensive capsule-making machines, which shorten this tedious process, is given in the resource section of this book, together with an address for purchasing capsules.

Most gelatine capsules are made from animal products, so vegetarians will not wish to use them. However capsules are probably the easiest way to take herbs and most patients take to them readily. Powdered herbs can be hard on a weak digestive system.

Pills

Pills are the main way commercial companies sell their herbal formulae. There are some rough and ready home pill-making techniques, such as rolling coarse-ground herbs into a dough made of moistened slippery elm powder or bread, and then letting this dry before cutting the hardened material up into 'pills'. But in my view, pill-making should be left to companies with the technical expertise and equipment.

Baths

Herbal baths have been an important method of treatment since ancient times. Luxuriating in a bath of hot herbal water encourages the pores of the skin to open, and allows the active principles of herbs to be absorbed directly into the body by osmosis. This method of treatment has been popularized by herbalists like Father Kneipp, and Maurice Mességué. For a full adult bath make up 4 litres of decoction and strain this before putting it into the bath. A weaker mixture can be made by tying a muslin bag full of herbs under the hot tap so that the hot water runs right through it. Hand and foot baths are also extremely effective. If you want to know more about this read Maurice Mességué's books (see the reading list). Herbal baths are particularly good for treating fractious children or teething babies – a chamomile or limeflower bath can often work wonders. Herbal baths can be made by simply dropping five or six drops of an essential oil into the bath. Lavender oil is relaxing, wintergreen or pine oil are good for aching muscles, and rosemary oil is a good pick-me-up. If using oils in a bath for children, dilute them in a vegetable oil first.

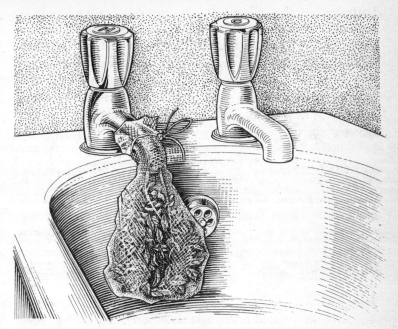

A muslin bag of herbs can be attached to the hot tap

Ointments

Ointments are one way to keep healing herbs in continuous contact with a diseased area of the body or skin. There are many ways to make ointments, and several considerations that need to be taken into account. For example, the greasier the base, the more it will prevent heat loss from inflamed skin. So a greasy ointment may not be ideal for treating acute eczema.

A simple soothing ointment can be made from fresh chickweed, sunflower oil and beeswax. Use a double boiler (bain-marie). Immerse 300 gm of chickweed in 480 ml of sunflower oil. Bring the water in the outer part of the double boiler to the boil, and simmer gently on a low heat for three to four hours, until the chickweed has lost its colour. Strain the oil and then re-heat it. Add 60 gm of beeswax and heat until melted. Add two drops of lavender oil for fragrance, and, to preserve the ointment, a drop of tincture of benzoin for each 30 ml of sunflower oil used.

A useful healing and drawing ointment can be made by melting together:

> Beeswax 60 gm
> Vegetable fat 360 gm

Macerate 240 gm of powdered marshmallow root in the ingredients over a low heat, for an hour. Take this off the heat and, when cool, using a spatula, mix in 150 gm of slippery-elm powder.

A soothing ointment can be made from the following:

> Elder flowers, dried 90 gm
> Red poppy flowers 90 gm

in a melted base of:
> White wax 150 gm
> Olive oil 450 ml

Macerate everything together for two hours. Strain and bottle.

Poultices

Using a poultice is another excellent way of applying herbs externally. Poultices are usually applied hot to relieve inflammation and promote blood circulation to a damaged area. Californian surgeons have recently measured the effect of heat treatment on the blood flow near wounds. They calculate that high temperatures increase the blood flow by three times the normal rate, so causing more oxygen to reach the wound, which helps to clear away harmful bacteria.

Poultices can be made from bread or many common vegetables. For a carrot poultice, boil organic carrots until soft and mash them to a pulp. Add a little olive oil to keep the carrots soft, and spread the pulped mass evenly between a double layer of cotton gauze. Lay the poultice on a sieve over the top of a pot of boiling water, allowing the steam to permeate it.

A similar poultice can be made using slippery-elm powder mixed with a strong infusion or decoction of herbs, to form a stiff paste. One of the most simple and effective poultices is made in just the same way, using coarse-ground comfrey root. A stimulating poultice uses:

> Crushed linseed 120 gm
> Mustard powder 8 gm
> Water 250 ml

Gradually add the linseed to the boiling water. Then add the mustard powder and stir. Spread this evenly on a double layer of cotton gauze. Take care to have a layer of gauze between the poultice and the skin, to avoid blistering. Be careful not to apply poultices too hot. For a good drawing action, poultices should be re-applied every ten to fifteen minutes, alternating two poultices, so that when one is in place, the other is being steam-heated. Cover poultices with a plastic bag to retain the heat as long as possible.

Compresses or fomentations

Compresses are a way of applying a decoction or infusion directly to the skin. A cloth is soaked in a hot, strained decoction and quickly wrung out before being placed on the skin. This is repeated, using two cloths alternately, to stimulate the area where the compress is applied.

Plasters

Medicated plasters are an under-rated method of local treatment, especially good for providing counter stimulation (e.g. using cayenne, wintergreen, thymol, etc) to treat rheumatic and muscular pains. They may also be used to heal damaged tissue (e.g. using marigold flowers). A plaster comprises these active herbal ingredients melted into a wax base, spread on to linen or butter muslin, which is then applied to the skin. The heat of the body softens the wax, and encourages the herbs to penetrate the skin.

Composing a prescription

Rules governing the putting together of a herbal prescription are not inscribed in tablets of stone. In fact, there is plenty of healthy argument amongst herbalists as to how this should be done. Some herbalists prefer, when making up their prescriptions, to use just one or two herbs at a time (single herbs are called 'simples'); other herbalists advocate mixing several herbs together in order to achieve the best effect. Certainly there is nothing to be said for a kind of 'shotgun prescribing', which sees a number of herbs thrown together in the hope that one or two will hit the target. At least if you get a result using a simple or single remedy, you know exactly what it was due to. But the systematic combining of herbs can greatly increase the efficacy of treatment. The idea of synergism – that two or more constituent parts of a plant can co-operate or support one another, to increase the effect of the whole plant – holds good for whole-plant mixtures too, when two or more plants can act as allies.

We find evidence for this in the fascinating work that has been done on companion planting. Experiments using the stinging nettle have shown that when it is grown alongside many herbs, it greatly increases their volatile oil content, yielding an increase of ten per cent in sage, twenty per cent in valerian and marjoram, nearly fifty per cent in peppermint, and an extraordinary eighty per cent in angelica. Companion planting has also shown that dandelions have a special affinity for alfalfa, and that rosemary and sage have a stimulating effect on one another.

More evidence in favour of plant combining comes from the discoveries of Dr E. E. Pfeiffer, who worked with Rudolf Steiner. Pfeiffer discovered that when a copper-chloride solution crystallizes on a glass plate, its tiny crystals form an irregular pattern. However if plant extracts are added to the crystallizing salt, then a co-ordinated pattern is produced. Moreover, each time the experiment is repeated, a particular plant will reproduce its characteristic pattern. A strong, healthy, vigorous plant will produce a clearly formed, harmonious crystal arrangement. But a crystallization made of a weak or diseased plant produces an uneven, disharmonious crystallization. These crystallization pictures have also been used to study the relationship between different plant species. This is done by mixing extracts of two plants in the copper-chloride solution. The new crystallization may show a stronger or weaker crystallization-picture, characteristic of one or other of the two plants used. This would indicate that one plant is either an ally (in the case of an enhanced crystal pattern), or antagonistic to the other (if the crystal pattern is weakened). Alternatively the crystallization-picture may show a balance of both plant 'signatures', in a harmonious and clearly formed pattern, which indicates a beneficial relationship between these two plants. One such experiment showed how equal extracts of peas and carrots together gave an integrated and harmonious mixture of the two original crystal pictures made by each plant on its own, so revealing mutual enhancement.[2] One of the two crystallization patterns shown here was produced with the juice from the plant greater celandine (*Chelidonium majus*). The other was produced with an extract of triturated gall-bladder. The striking similarity between them is said to demonstrate the specific relationship between greater celandine and the gallbladder. In fact, greater celandine has an ancient reputation for treating diseases of the gall-bladder. More research needs to be done on the compatibility, or otherwise, of herbal medicines, using this technique.

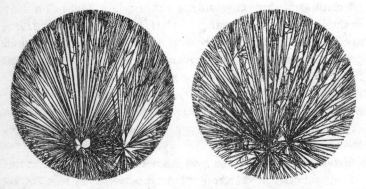

Root of Greater celandine pattern, Gallbladder pattern

Plant combining is a fundamental feature of traditional Chinese herbal medicine. Every formula is built on the understanding that one herb can help another. The interaction of herbs in prescriptions is discussed in the *Shanghan Lun* (*Discussion of Cold-induced Disorders*). Some examples of the categories it outlines give the general idea.

Mutual enhancement

Here two substances with a similar function are combined mutually to enhance and accentuate their overall action.

One such famous Chinese combination is that of rhubarb and glauber's salt, both of which have a cold nature and a purgative action. In western herbalism, a similar mutual accentuation occurs by combining the two heart tonics lily of the valley and hawthorn.

Mutual assistance

In this case two herbs, having essentially different functions and natures, are used together to enhance the effect of one of them when treating a specific problem. Through such mutual assistance, oedema (a build-up of fluid in the tissues) can be treated by using the diuretic herb poria together with astragalus, the famous Chinese energy (Qi) tonic.

Mutual counteraction

Herbs can be combined to reduce an unwanted side-effect of one of them. Thus, pinellia, a frequently used Chinese herb – which in its raw state is mildly poisonous, producing a dry mouth and heart palpitations – is rendered completely safe by being cooked with fresh ginger. In western herbalism, purgatives like senna and cascara are generally combined with aromatic herbs, like mint and ginger, to prevent griping.

Mutual incompatibility

Mutual incompatibility occurs when herbs which on their own are beneficial are combined and give unwanted side effects. Traditional Chinese herbal texts warn, for instance, against combining liquorice with a particular kind of seaweed (*Sargassum fusiforme*).

These general principles about combining different herbs formed the basis of a flexible framework for constructing traditional Chinese herbal prescriptions. The ideas are expressed in pre-Communist, feudal terms, which were seen to be a mirror of universal structures or laws. Thus most Chinese prescriptions contain one or more herbs that fulfil the function of the Sovereign, Minister, Assistant and Messenger.

The Sovereign is the principal ingredient which gives the prescription its main overall therapeutic effect. *The Minister* helps or enhances the effect of the Sovereign herb. *The Assistant* may either act to treat a secondary aspect, which is being treated simultaneously with the main one, or may moderate the harshness of the primary herbs, so helping the Sovereign and Minister herbs do their work. *The Messenger* directs the prescription as a whole to certain energy channels, areas of the body or organs. Messenger herbs may also have an overall harmonizing effect on the prescription. Liquorice is often used like this by both Chinese and western trained herbalists. For an analysis of a prescription along these lines see Appendix B.

The American physiomedical herbalists also thought that herb combinations would improve therapeutic results. Dr Lyle, to whom we have already referred, wrote:

Many agents having a general influence over the structures will expand their force – either where most needed, or in the directions whither they may be influenced by other medicines. Lobelia combined with honey or sugar, which are expectorants, will mostly influence the lungs and bronchii, and is an expectorant. Lobelia with laxatives will assist in producing catharsis ... Hydrastis is a very fine tonic to the stomach, but when combined with diuretics, it will tone the renal organs; with hepatics it will tone the liver and portal circulation ...[3]

I conclude by saying that although the use of 'simples' certainly has its place, the majority of clinical problems are best treated by carefully combining herbs according to these principles. This is the area where herbalists are like good cooks, skilfully blending their ingredients together to harmonize the whole in an effective 'recipe'.

APPENDIX A

HOLISM AND SCIENCE

The mechanistic view expounded by Descartes and Isaac Newton dominated scientific thinking from the second half of the seventeenth century until the first field theory proposed by Michael Faraday and Clerk Maxwell who, in the nineteenth century, investigated the nature of electric and magnetic forces. In the twentieth century new and revolutionary ideas about the way in which the universe works have been put forward by physicists. In formulating the quantum theory, they have effectively dismantled the Newtonian model of the universe, or rather have shown that it is, at best, only a partial glimpse of reality. Physicist David Bohm gives us some idea of the extraordinary shift of perspective brought about by the new physics:

One is led to a new notion of unbroken wholeness, which denies the classical idea of analyzability of the world into separately and independently existing parts . . . We have reversed the usual classical notion that the independent 'elementary parts' of the world are the fundamental reality, and that the various systems are merely particular contingent forms and arrangements of these parts. Rather we say that inseparable quantum interconnectedness of the whole universe is the fundamental reality, and that relatively independently behaving parts are merely particular and contingent forms within this whole.[1]

Biologists have been rather slower than the physicists to accept that an exclusively mechanistic view may have its limitations. The modern discovery of DNA and the breaking of its genetic code have seemed to confirm the essentially mechanical nature of life and the validity of mechanistic techniques to make all future discoveries. Yet despite these, and other remarkable discoveries made by analytical techniques and a separation of parts, a more holistic view amongst biologists has refused to lie down and die. Indeed, with the 1981 publication of his highly controversial book *A New Science of Life*, Rupert Sheldrake has resurrected it with some gusto. Dr Sheldrake acknowledges the holistic tradition in biology to which he is heir:

There has always been, within biology, an holistic tradition that has tried to understand the nature of living things in a different way. The holistic tradition historically grows out of the vitalist tradition, and the vitalist tradition has grown from the Aristotelian and Scholastic traditions. The basic idea here is that living organisms – or indeed, nature – are *self-organizing*; i.e. they have their own purposes, their own goals, their own ability to organize themselves. For Aristotle and the scholastics of the Middle Ages, this organizing principle was called the *psyche* or *soul*. Their concept of soul was rather different from the vague and confused ideas that are common today, which confine it to human beings. The psyche or soul was present in all living things – animals, plants and, indeed, the whole earth – and was also, as Aristotle (and also Plato) puts it, the form of the body. The soul was not in the body, the body was in the soul; it was this which shaped and formed the body . . .[2]

Dr Sheldrake is concerned with a central question in biology, which is how plants and animals attain their form. Form cannot be represented mathematically, nor through biochemical analysis, yet it is the characteristic feature of all living organisms. After all, do we not classify all flora and fauna by their shape and form? Because of evident difficulties in existing theories, Sheldrake sought a new hypothesis to explain how life attains its form. He asked the classical mechanistic biologists how DNA, which is exactly the same in every single cell of the body, can instruct the various structures of the body like the eyes, ears or brain, to develop in their own characteristic way. Sheldrake explained how embryologists, in an attempt to come to grips with the problem of form in the 1920s, came up with the concept of *morphogenetic fields*. The word morphogenetic is derived from two Greek words – *morphe* (shape or form), and *genesis* (birth or origin). Morphogenetic fields were presumed in and around an embryo, as its organizing force. This idea was not so revolutionary as it might at first appear; modern physics had already established that there was no fundamental difference between space and matter, as Fritjof Capra so clearly explains:

The field theories of modern physics force us to abandon the classical distinction between material particles and the void. Einstein's field theory of gravity and his quantum field theory both show that particles cannot be separated from the space surrounding them. On the one hand, they determine the structure of that space; on the other hand they cannot be regarded as isolated entities, but have to be seen as condensations of a continuous field which is present throughout space ... The discovery of the dynamic quality of the vacuum is seen by many physicists as one of the most important findings of modern physics. From its role as an empty container of the physical phenomena, the void has emerged as a dynamic quantity of the utmost importance.[3]

According to Dr Sheldrake, the concept of morphogenetic fields provides a way for us to understand how, if a flatworm is cut up into several pieces, each part can regenerate to make another whole worm; and how, from a single cutting, a whole new tree – roots, trunk, branches and leaves – might grow. This property of wholeness, Sheldrake explains, is a phenomenon of fields. He gives as an example the observation that if you cut a magnet into small bits, you get several smaller magnets, each with its own magnetic field intact. Yet until the publication of Sheldrake's book, it seemed that this concept of morphogenetic fields was to remain deliberately vague, many biologists regarding them as merely a useful idea, but with no basis in reality. Sheldrake's bold step was to suggest that morphogenetic fields do exist in reality, just like electrical and gravitational fields. Morphogenetic fields, he holds, are responsible for the characteristic form and shape of all matter, whether living or not, and these fields are connected to, and influenced by, what has happened in the past:

The morphogenetic fields of all past systems become *present* to any subsequent similar system; the structures of past systems affect subsequent similar systems by a cumulative influence which acts across both space *and time*.[4]

From the herbalist's point of view the concept of morphogenetic fields helps to underpin the concept of vital force (*vis medicatrix naturae*). Dr Sheldrake's hypothesis also irons out a distinction between the western concept of vital force and the eastern idea of Qi. As it is often used by vitalists, the notion of vital force is essentially dualistic, assuming some non-physical arbiter of form acting upon the physical. Sheldrake's ideas about morphogenetic fields avoid such a dualistic thinking:

... morphogenetic fields are spatial structures, detectable only through their morphogenetic effects on material systems; they ... can be regarded as aspects of matter if the definition of matter is widened still further to include them.[5] *

* Rupert Sheldrake's ideas also bear resemblance to the Chinese concept *Li*, as explained by the brilliant Chinese philosopher Wang Pi: 'Things do not struggle among themselves at random. They flow of necessity from their principles of order (*Li*). They are integrated by a root cause. They are gathered together by a single influence. Thus things are complex but not chaotic. There is multiplicity of them, but not confusion.'

The eminent Chinese scholar, Joseph Needham, comments on Wang Pi's conception of *Li*: 'What he was trying to describe was perhaps a series of fields of force (as we might call them), contained in, but subsidiary to, the main field of the force of the Tao, and each manifesting itself at different points in space and time'.[6]

This accords with the Chinese idea of Qi, which sees no duality between matter and energy, for matter is nothing but condensed Qi in another form. As the famous neo-Confucian philosopher Chang Tsai wrote:

When the Qi condenses, its visibility becomes apparent, so that there are the shapes (of individual things). When it disperses, its visibility is no longer apparent and there are no shapes.[7]

An idea echoed by the Taoist Chuang Tzu:

Man's life is due to the conglomeration of the Qi, and when they are dispersed, death occurs . . . Therefore it is said that all through the universe there is one Qi, and therefore sages prized that unity.[8]

CHINESE MEDICINE:

PRINCIPLES, PRESCRIPTIONS

AND ANALYSIS

The Eight Principles

Traditional Chinese herbal doctors (and acupuncturists) collect information about the patient by four methods: looking (including tongue diagnosis), asking, listening/smelling, and touching (which includes pulse diagnosis). The signs and symptoms that are collected are classified and measured according to eight principles (listed below), and by consideration of the special characteristics of the internal organs (*Zhang-fu*), such as those of the spleen and stomach described in the footnote on page 71, as well as the special characteristics of the channels and collaterals (*Jing luo*). In this manner complex clinical problems can be understood in a systematic way.

The eight principles are actually four pairs of opposites.

Yin	Yang
Interior	Exterior
Deficiency	Excess
Cold	Hot

The main division is that of yin and yang. The other three pairs of opposites are a means of defining what kind of yin or yang imbalance has occurred. These eight principles are the tool by which the doctor can establish, in a general way, the location, temperature and strength of a disease. The category interior/exterior tells of the depth of the disease; the category hot/cold tells about the nature of disease; that of excess/deficiency tells of the virulence of the disease versus the resilience of the body; and the yin/yang category tells about the overall nature of the pattern of disharmony.

Since this is not a textbook on Chinese medicine, we will not discuss these categories in any detail here. For a full exposition of the eight principles, and other aspects of Chinese diagnosis, see Ted Kaptchuk's *Chinese Medicine*, published by Rider and Co. in 1983.

Analysis according to traditional hierarchy

Cinnamon Twig Soup (*Gui Zhi Tang*)

Cinnamon Twig Soup is one of the most famous Chinese herbal prescriptions, dating back to the *Shang-han Lun* (*Discussion of Cold-induced Disorders*). It consists of five herbs:

> Cinnamon twigs (*Cinnamonum cassia*)
> White peony root (*Paeonia lactiflora*)
> Fresh ginger (*Zingiber officinale*)
> Chinese dates (*Ziziphus jujuba*)
> Honey-baked liquorice (*Glycyrrhiza uralensis*)

This prescription is often used in the first and most external of the six stages of disease (*Tai Yang* or Greater Yang), provoked by the attack of wind-cold 'evil'. Typical signs and symptoms in such a case would be headache, fever with chills, aches and pains (especially in the shoulders and back of the neck), runny nose, sore throat, dislike of draughts, and possibly some sweating due to the attack by wind, which damages the ability of the pores to close. In fact, Cinnamon Twig Soup is particularly appropriate when there is *ineffective* sweating, which fails to clear the wind-cold evil.

In this prescription the **Sovereign** herb is cinnamon twig, which is acrid, sweet and warm. This herb is used to ward off attacks of wind-cold. On its own, cinnamon twig provokes sweating. It has a strongly yang nature and strengthens the yang defensive Qi (*Wei Qi*), which flows in the superficial (*yang*) aspect of the body. (It is interesting that the outer part of the cinnamon tree, the twigs, strengthen the outer energies of the human body, while the inner bark of the tree strengthens the deeper yang activity of the kidney and spleen. Here we have a subtle doctrine of signatures, which is often apparent in herbal medicine. The Chinese teach that in general roots treat interior disease, while the nature of flowers is to lift and float, so many flower remedies are used to treat exterior disease. Climbing plants, it is said, are good for treating channel disease, seeds have a sinking nature, and so on. However, the Chinese are highly pragmatic and never allow a general theory to impose itself on actual clinical observation. In other words, there are some exceptions to this principle.)

The **Minister** herb is white peony root, which is bitter, sour and cool. Although white peony is often used to nourish the blood or to calm disrupted liver Qi, it also has the capacity to gather the yin and harmonize the nutritive or deeper Qi (*Ying Qi*), and so can be used to stop sweating. Where there is ineffective sweating, white peony is often combined with cinnamon twigs, which, as we have seen, strengthen the external defensive Qi. White peony has a yin nature; cinnamon twigs a yang nature. The two herbs work in harmony together: the cinnamon twigs – or Sovereign – going to the outside (dispersing); the peony – or Minister – to the inside (gathering). Both herbs work at harmonizing and strengthening the

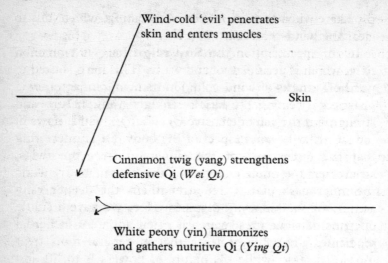

Wind-cold 'evil' penetrates
skin and enters muscles

Skin

Cinnamon twig (yang) strengthens
defensive Qi (*Wei Qi*)

White peony (yin) harmonizes
and gathers nutritive Qi (*Ying Qi*)

body's energy in order to expel the wind-cold (see diagram).

The **Assistant** consists of two herbs – ginger and Chinese dates. Ginger is acrid, hot and causes sweating, so that it acts to reinforce the therapeutic effects of cinnamon twig in dispelling, from the superficial level of the body, a wind-cold 'evil'. Its combination with Chinese dates, which are sweet and neutral in nature, echoes in minor key the more potent combination of cinnamon twig and peony; Chinese dates, like white peony, also act to adjust the inner, nutritive Qi (*Ying Qi*). The dates also play a valuable role in protecting the digestive system against possible damage from the hot acrid herbs – ginger and cinnamon.

The **Messenger** is honey-baked liquorice. Liquorice, when baked, is sweet and slightly warm (when raw it has a cool nature). It is included in an enormous number of Chinese prescriptions because it harmonizes, unifies and moderates the actions of other herbs, making powerful herbs like cinnamon more gentle. It is an effective Messenger, for the Chinese say that it enters all twelve primary channels or meridians, and can lead other herbs with which it is combined, throughout the body. Honey-baked liquorice is generally thought kinder on the digestion, so in this respect it mirrors the activity of the Chinese dates.

If there is an attack of wind-cold 'evil' in which there is no sweating, then an altogether different prescription is appropriate. Because the main requirement here is to open the pores and stimulate sweating, the alternative prescription is the Soup of Ma Huang (*Ma Huang Tang*). This prescription uses ma huang (which is a stronger diaphoretic than cinnamon) as the Sovereign herb, while cinnamon twig fulfils the function of Minister.

Three Chinese herbal prescriptions

1 *White Tiger Soup* (*Bai hu tang*)

This prescription, taken from the *Shang-han Lun*, has four ingredients:

> Gypsum (*Calcium sulphate*)
> Amenarrhena (*Amenarrhena asphodeloides*)
> Honey-baked liquorice (*Glycyrrhiza uralensis*)
> Rice (*Oryza sativa*)

Its purpose is to eliminate heat from the Qi stage of the four stages – *Wei*, *Qi*, *Ying* and *Blood*. Here the external 'evil' has not been dispelled from the *Wei*, or outer portion of the body, and drives deeper inwards.

White Tiger soup also deals with disease which has penetrated to the *Yang Ming* (Yang Brightness) level, according to the earlier six-stage scheme of disease progression devised by Zhang Zhong-jing. Here the external 'evil' has broken through the first, *Tai Yang* (Greater Yang) stage (characterized by a dislike of wind and cold, headache, stuffy nose and a floating pulse). Although Zhang Zhong-jing counted the *Yang Ming* stage as the second of his six stages, this should by rights be the *Shao Yang* (Lesser Yang) stage, since this *Shao Yang* stage describes that time when an 'evil' is neither superficial (as in the *Tai Yang* stage) nor inside (as in the *Yang Ming* stage). However, in devising this system, Zhang Zhong-jing took his cue from a passage in the Yellow Emperor's *Classic of Internal Medicine* (*Huang-di Nei-Jing*), which describes how a cold 'evil', on the first day of entering the body, injures the *Tai Yang*; on the second day it damages the *Yang Ming*; on the third day, the *Shao Yang*; and so on, going deeper and deeper into the body.

The White Tiger Soup prescription promotes the secretion of body fluids and cools out the fever.

Apart from the diagnostic signs already mentioned in the text, the tongue-body typically is red, having a dry, yellow coating. The pulse is rapid, forceful or slippery. If the pulse is weak, then **ginseng** (*Panax ginseng*) is a common addition to this prescriptive formula, since it tonifies the body's Qi and helps it overcome the external evil.

Gypsum is pungent, sweet and very cold. It clears stomach fire and relieves thirst. **Amenarrhena** is bitter and cold. It clears heat from the lungs and stomach. It moistens and nourishes the yin of the body and so prevents the body fluids from being damaged by fever. **Honey-baked liquorice** is sweet and neutral. It harmonizes the whole prescription and tonifies the spleen. **Rice** is also sweet and neutral. It helps to moisten the stomach and revive the spleen (i.e. the digestion as a whole).

2 The Schizonepeta-ledebouriella Defeating Poisons Powder (Jing-fang Bai-du San)

This prescription comprises eleven herbs:

> Schizonepeta (*Schizonepeta tenuifolia*)
> Ledebouriella (*Ledebouriella seseloides*)
> Bupleurum (*Bupleurum scorzoneraefolium*)
> Chinese lovage (*Ligusticum wallichii*)
> Notopterygium (*Notopterygium incisium*)
> Pubescent angelica (*Angelica pubescens*)
> Tangerine peel (*Citrus reticulata*)
> Balloonflower root (*Platycodon grandiflorum*)
> Hogfennel root (*Peucedanum praeruptorum*)
> Tuckahoe (*Poria cocos*)
> Liquorice (*Glycyrrhiza uralensis*)

Schizonepeta, ledebouriella and **bupleurum** cause sweating, free the exterior, and drive out the cold. **Chinese lovage, notopterygium** and **pubescent angelica** drive out the wind and any associated dampness (another common external 'evil'). The five other herbs in this prescription – **tangerine peel, balloonflower root, hogfennel root, tuckahoe** and **liquorice** – resolve phlegm, strengthen the Qi and the lungs. The lungs are the organs which govern the body's defensive Qi (*Wei Qi*); they are usually the first organ to be affected by an external 'evil'.

3 The Honeysuckle-forsythia Powder (Yin-qiao San)

This prescription is made up of ten herbs:

> Honeysuckle flowers (*Lonicera japonica*)
> Forsythia (*Forsythia suspensa*)
> Schizonepeta (*Schizonepeta tenuifolia*)
> Mint (*Mentha arvensis*)
> Prepared soya bean (*Glycine max*)
> Balloonflower (*Platycodon grandiflorum*)
> Burdock seed (*Arctium lappa*)

Liquorice (*Glycyrrhiza uralensis*)
Reed rhizome (*Phragmites communis*)
Bamboo leaf (*Phyllostachys nigra*)

Schizonepeta, mint and **prepared soya bean** have an effect of cooling and reducing heat. **Forsythia** and **honeysuckle** also act in this way, and have the further application of being anti-bacterial and anti-viral. **Balloonflower, burdock seed** and **liquorice** clear congestion and phlegm from the lungs and soothe a sore throat. **Reed rhizome** and **bamboo leaf** cool and reduce heat, moisten dryness and calm the nervous system.

NOTES

Introduction

1. Dr William Court, 'Pulse Reference', *Pulse*, 20 Oct 1984.
2. Eric Block, 'The Chemistry of Garlic and Onions', *Scientific American*, March 1985.
3. J. D. Phillipson and L. Anderson, 'Herbal Remedies used in Sedative and Anti-rheumatic Preparations', *Pharmaceutical Journal*, 28 July 1984.
4. Professor Vano E. Tyler, 'Plant Drugs in the Twenty-first Century', *Economic Botany*, June 1986.
5. *Herbalgram*, No. 11, Winter 1987.
6. Steven Fulder, *The Root of Being*, Hutchinson, 1980.
7. Beryl Rowland (tr.), *Mediaeval Women's Guide to Health*, Kent State University Press and Croom Helm Ltd, 1981.

Chapter One

1. R. H. Charles (tr), *The Book of Enoch*, SPCK, 1917.
2. William Withering, *An Account of the Foxglove and Some of Its Uses*, Longwood Press, 1977 (reprint of 1785 ed.).
3. Sir Wallis Budge's discussion of the *Ebers Papyrus* in *The Divine Origin of the Craft of the Herbalist*, Society of Herbalists, 1928.
4. Ibid.
5. *Oncology*, Vol. 43, pp. 93–7, 1986.
6. Packard, 'Gui Patin and the Medical Profession in Paris in the Seventeenth Century', *AMH*, IV, no. 3, pp. 215–216, (quoted by Barbara Griggs, *Green Pharmacy*, Hobhouse, 1981).
7. B. Griggs, *Green Pharmacy*, Hobhouse, 1981.
8. J. Jacobi (ed.), *Paracelsus: Selected Writings* (2nd edn.), p. 169, Princetown University Press, 1958.

Chapter Two

1. Report by Boyce Rensberger, *International Herald Tribune*, 2 January 1986.
2. Richard Grossinger, *Planet Medicine: From Stone Age Shamanism to Post Industrial Healing*, Shambhala Publications, 1982.
3. Carlos Castaneda, *The Fire from Within*, Century, 1985.
4. Richard Evans Schultes and Albert Hoffman, *Plants of the Gods*, Hutchinson, 1980.
5. Ibid.
6. David Hoffman, *The Holistic Herbal*, Findhorn Press, 1983.
7. J. E. Lovelock, *Gaia*, OUP, 1979.
8. Oliver Sacks, *The Man who Mistook his Wife for a Hat*, Picador, 1985.
9. Hippocrates, *The Nature of Man*, see Jones, W. H. S. (ed. and tr), *Hippocrates with an English Translation*, 1–4, Harvard University Press, 1931, 1952.
10. René Descartes, *Discourse on Method and the Meditations*, Penguin, 1987.
11. Joseph Needham, *Science and Civilization in China*, II, p. 369, CUP, 1954.
12. Ilza Veith (tr.), *The Yellow Emperor's Classic of Internal Medicine*, University of California Press, 1972.
13. J. Jacobi (ed.), *Paracelsus: Selected Writings* (2nd ed.), Princetown University Press, 1958.
14. John Skelton, *The Science and Practice of Medicine*, John Skelton, MRSC, 1904.
15. W. H. Cook, *Science and Practice of Medicine*, Cincinnati, 1879.
16. Research carried out by Dr Stewart Johnson, City of London Migraine Clinic. See his book *Feverfew*, Sheldon Press, 1984.
17. John Parkinson, *Theatrum Botanicum*, 1640, available from the Bodleian Library, Oxford.
18. John Hill, *The Family Herbal*, 1772, available from the Bodleian Library.

19. Dr William A. R. Thomson quoted by Robert Eagle in *Alternative Medicine*, Futura, 1978.
20. Dr William A. R. Thomson, *Healing Plants*, Macmillan, 1978.
21. Dr William Court, Lecture at First International Conference of Herbal Medicine, London, 1985.

Chapter Three

1. J. H. Gaddum, *Pharmacology*, p. 167, OUP, 1959.
2. Colin Tudge, *Guardian*, 2 January 1987.
3. W. H. Cook, *Science and Practice of Medicine*, Black Swan Books, Cincinnati, 1879.
4. Ibid.
5. Dr T. J. Lyle, *Physiomedical Therapeutics: Materia Medica and Pharmacy*, originally published Ohio 1897, republished 1932, by the National Association of Medical Herbalists, London.
6. Unpublished material, translated by Richard Temple.

Chapter Four

1. Dr T. J. Lyle, op. cit.

Chapter Seven

1. J. M. Thurston, *The Philosophy of Physiomedicalism*, Richmond, Indiana, 1900.
2. H. Philbrick and R. B. Gregg, *Companion Plants*, Watkins, 1977.
3. Dr T. J. Lyle, op. cit.

Appendix A

1. D. Bohm and B. Hiley, 'On the Intuitive Understanding of Nonlocality as Implied by Quantum Theory', *Foundations of Physics*, Vol. 5, 1975. Quoted by Fritjof Capra, *The Tao of Physics*, Fontana, 1976.

2. An extract from a seminar given by Rupert Sheldrake: 'The Presence of the Past', *Beshara*, Vol. 1, Spring 1987.
3. Fritjof Capra, *The Tao of Physics*, Fontana, 1976.
4. Rupert Sheldrake, *A New Science of Life*, Paladin, 1987.
5. Ibid.
6. Joseph Needham, *Science and Civilisation in China*, Vol. II, CUP, 1956.
7. Originally quoted in Fung Yu-lan's *A Short History of Chinese Philosophy*, Macmillan, New York, 1958.
8. Joseph Needham, op. cit.

FURTHER READING

This list comprises those books from the many about herbal medicine currently published, I have found useful.

Buchman, Dian, *Herbal Medicine*, Herb Society & Rider & Co., 1983.

Campion, Kitty, *Handbook of Herbal Health*, Sphere, 1985.

Chardenon, Ludo, *In Praise of Wild Herbs*, Century, 1985.

Christopher, Dr John, *School of Natural Healing*, Biworld Publishers, 1976.

Culpeper, Nicholas, *The Complete Herbal*, Wehman, 1960.

Ellingwood, Finley, *American Materia Medica: Therapeutics and Pharmacognosy*, Eclectic Medical Publications, 1983.

Gerard, John, *The Herbal*, Dover, 1975.

Gosling, Nalda, *Successful Herbal Remedies*, Thorsons, 1985.

Grieve, Mrs M., *A Modern Herbal*, Penguin, 1976.

Griggs, Barbara, *Green Pharmacy*, Hobhouse, 1981.

Hoffmann, David, *The Holistic Herbal*, Findhom Press, 1983.
The Herb User's Guide, Thorsons, 1987.

Lust, John, *The Herb Book*, Bantam, 1974.

Maybe R., and McIntyre M., *The New Herbalist*, Elm Tree, 1988.

McIntyre, Anne, *Herbs for Pregnancy and Childbirth*, Sheldon Press, 1988.

Mességué, Maurice, *Health Secrets of Plants and Herbs*, Collins, 1979.
Of Men and Plants, Macmillan, 1974.
Way to Natural Health and Beauty, Allen & Unwin, 1976.

Mills, Simon, *The Dictionary of Modern Herbalism*, Thorsons, 1985.

Palaiseul, Jean, *Grandmother's Secrets*, Penguin, 1976.

Priest, A. W., and Priest, L. R., *Herbal Medication*, Fowler, 1982.

Roberts, Frank, *Modern Herbalism for Digestive Disorders*, Thorsons, 1978.

Schauenburg, Paul, and Paris, Ferdinand, *Guide to Medicinal Plants*, Lutterworth Press, 1977.

Smith, William, *Wonders in Weeds*, Health Science Press, 1977.

Stuart, Malcolm (ed.), *The Encyclopedia of Herbs and Herbalism*, Guild Publishing, 1986.

Thomson, William A. R., *Healing Plants*, Macmillan, 1978.

Tiera, Michael, *The Way of Herbs*, Unity Press, 1982.

Valnet, Dr Jean, *Phytotherapie*, Maloine, 1979.

Vogel, J., *American Indian Medicine*, University of Oklahoma Press, 1970.

Chinese Herbal Medicine

Bensky, Dan, and Gamble, Andrew, *Chinese Herbal Medicine and Materia Medica*, Eastland Press, 1986.

Kaptchuk, Ted, *Chinese Medicine*, Rider & Co., 1983.

Keys, John, *Chinese Herbs*, Charles Tuttle & Co., 1976.

Teeguarden, R., *Chinese Tonic Herbs*, Japan Publications, 1985.

Yeung, Him-che, *Handbook of Chinese Herbs and Formulas*, Los Angeles, 1985.

Ayurvedic Medicine

Lad, Dr Vasant, *Ayurveda: The Science of Self Healing*, Lotus Press, 1984.

Lad, Dr Vasant, and Frawley, David, *The Yoga of Herbs*, Lotus Press, 1986.

Tibetan Medicine

Burang, Theodore, *Tibetan Art of Healing*, Watkins, 1974.

Donden, Dr Yeshi, *Health Through Balance*, Snow Lion Publications, 1986.

USEFUL ADDRESSES

Wholesale Herbal Suppliers

Brome and Schimmer Ltd
Unit 3
Romsey Industrial Estate
Romsey
Hants SO51 0HR

Cathay of Bournemouth Ltd
Hampshire House
Bourne Avenue
Bournemouth BH2 6DW

East-West Herbs (Chinese and Western Herb Stock)
Langston Priory Mews
Kingham
Oxon OX7 6UW

Frank Roberts (Herbal Dispensaries) Ltd
91 Newfoundland Road
Bristol
Avon BS2 9LT

Gerard House Ltd
3 Wickham Road
Boscomb
Bournemouth BH7 6JX

The Herbal Apothecary
50 The Half Croft
Syston
Leicester LE7 8LD

Phytoproducts
Tidebrook Manor Farm
Wadhurst
Sussex TN5 6PD

Pierce Arnold and Son
Pollard Road
Morden
Surrey SM4 6EG

Potters Herbal Supplies Ltd
Leyland Mill Lane
Wigan
Lancs WN1 2SB

Weleda UK Ltd (also Homeopathic medicines)
Heanor Road
Ilkeston
Derbyshire DE7 8DR

Retail Herbal Suppliers

G. Baldwins & Co.
171–173 Walworth Road
London SE17

Dr Edward Bach Centre (Bach Flower Remedies)
Mount Vernon
Sotwell
Wallingford
Oxon OX10 0PZ

Napier of Edinburgh (also some wholesale)
18 Bristol Place
Edinburgh EH1 1HA

Neal's Yard Apothecary
2 Neal's Yard
Covent Garden
London WC2

Herbal Tinctures and Fluid Extracts

Fluid extracts are supplied by Potters Herbal Supplies Ltd
Tinctures are supplied by: East-West Herbs
                          The Herbal Apothecary
                          Phytoproducts
for addresses see above list

Capsule-Filling Machines

These are supplied by East-West Herbs (see above) or
Davcaps
PO Box 11
Monmouth
Gwent NP5 3NX
Gelatine capsules are also supplied by Davcaps.

Training

The only full-time course is run by
The School of Herbal Medicine/Phytotherapy
148 Forest Road
Tunbridge Wells
Kent TN2 5EY

Other courses

The School of Herbal Medicine/Phytotherapy

Dr Christopher's School of Natural Healing
19 Park Terrace
Stoke on Trent
Staffs

School of Natural Medicine
Dolphin House
6 Gold Street
Saffron Walden
Essex CB10 IEJ

The General Council and Register of Consultant Herbalists Ltd
Malborough House
Swanpool
Falmouth
Cornwall TR11 4HW

The School of Chinese Herbal Medicine
Pine Trees
Chiltern Road
Amersham
Bucks HP6 5PG

Other Useful Addresses

National Institute of Medical Herbalists
41 Hatherley Road
Winchester
Hants SO22 6RR

British Herbal Medicine Association
The Old Coach House
Southborough Road
Surbiton
Surrey

The Register of Chinese Herbal Medicine
7a Stanhope Road
London N6 5NE

The British Herb Grower's Association
17 Hooker Street
London SW3

Herb Society
77 Great Peter Street
London SW1P 2EZ

Suffolk Herbs Ltd
Sawyers Farm
Little Cornard
Sudbury
Suffolk CO10 0NY

USA

American Herb Association
Box 353
Rescue CA96 672

Mark Blumenthal
Herbalgram (an excellent journal)
PO Box 12602
Austin
Texas 78711

Herb Research Foundation
Box 2602
Longmont CO80501

Australia

National Herbalists Association of Australia
49 Oakwood Street
Sutherland
New South Wales 2232

INDEX